animaLs anD
psycHeDeLics

ANIMALS AND PSYCHEDELICS

The Natural World and the Instinct to Alter Consciousness

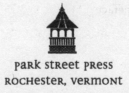

GIORGIO SAMORINI
TRANSLATED BY TAMI CALLIOPE

PARK STREET PRESS
ROCHESTER, VERMONT

Park Street Press
One Park Street
Rochester, Vermont 05767
www.InnerTraditions.com

Park Street Press is a division of Inner Traditions International

Originally published in Italian under the title *Animali che si drogano*
by Telesterion Vicenza
Copyright © 2000 by Telesterion Vicenza
English translation copyright © 2002 by Inner Traditions

Library of Congress Cataloging-in-Publication Data
Samorini, Giorgio, 1957-
[Animali che si drogano. English]
Animals and psychedelics : the natural world and the instinct
to alter consciousness / Giorgio Samorini ; translated by Tami
Calliope; foreword by Robert Montgomery.
  p. cm.
Includes bibliographical references.
 ISBN 978-0-89281-986-7
 1. Animals—Drug use. I. Title.
 QL756.7 .S26 2002
 591.5—dc21

                                        2002000622

Printed and bound in the United States

10 9 8 7 6 5 4

Text design and layout by Mary Anne Hurhula
This book was typeset in Cochin with Disturbance
as the display typeface

contents

Foreword
Evolution Through Inebriation?   vii

Introduction
Drugs in the Animal Kingdom and Beyond   1

1 Crazed Cows   18

2 Alcohol and Animals:
From Drunken Elephants to
Sauced Snails   27

3 Frenzied Felines   32

4 Mushroom-Loving Reindeer
and Craving Caribou   38

5 Galloping Goats   43

6 Birds on a Binge   48

7 Other "Out There" Animals   55

8 Intoxicated Insects   62

9 The Lazarus Fly: A New Hypothesis   68

10 Animals, Humans, and Drugs:
    The Why of It All   76

References   89
Index   94

Foreword

EVOLUTION THROUGH INEBRIATION?

That animals drug themselves is a deceptively simple statement. Contained within it, as within the pages of this remarkable book, is nothing short of a radical reexamination of what it is to be human. The consequences of this simple truth are both far reaching and immediate.

Let's begin by breaking this concept down into two aspects: first, that animals do drug themselves as a nonartificial impulse and second, that they do so intentionally. That they *drug* themselves requires drawing upon the comparatively precise sciences of botany, chemistry, and pharmacology to discover what exactly are the drug sources, their composition, and their activity. That animals drug *themselves* raises a different order of consideration. This involves the scientific study of animal behavior, or ethology. Although it may be possible to know through behavioral observation whether an animal is intoxicated or not, and by what means, some of the more subtle—and therefore most intriguing—types of altered states and inebriation can be difficult to discern. Much less can be understood about the nature of that animal's felt experience, let alone what the individual's motivation might be for consuming the drug. This field of study, however, promises such fascinating and crucial insights into the nature of consciousness that we are compelled to explore it with every resource available. The results will surprise you.

We all are familiar with neighborhood cats indulging themselves with garden catnip, and many know about the pet monkeys that enjoy smoking tobacco cigarettes. Most of us have heard of animals in cruel laboratory research clinics self-administering drugs such as cocaine. We can even conjure images of animals, on their own, unwittingly consuming fermented fruits or psychoactive plants and experiencing accidental intoxication. But how many of us realize that—entirely on their own and without the influence of captivity or conditioning—wild animals, birds, and even insects do indeed drug themselves? This deliberate seeking of inebriation among all classes of animals is a perfectly natural, normative behavior. Indeed, the pursuit of inebriation has been proposed as a kind of fourth drive—akin to hunger, thirst, and sex—so ubiquitous is its manifestation.

Animals engage in intoxicating drug consumption. This fact forms one of the most provocative and original of Giorgio Samorini's insights: this moment of drug-induced inebriation produces a *deschematizzazione*, or deconditioning, that allows for new behavioral ways to be established in a species. This prefaces the long-established discovery by R. Gordon Wasson and successive others, that consciousness-expanding plants and mushrooms are key to the origins of humanity itself and the inspiration for religious thought, influencing humanity since remotest history through the present and surely into our future. Before taking this conceptual leap from the influence of psychoactive drugs on human culture to their influence on species evolution, we must ask what distinguishes human from animal awareness, and is it such a great distinction at all?

Ethology is the science of animal behavior, ethnobotany studies human uses for plants, and ethnopharmacognosy is the science of human use of *drug* plants.

Ethno*zöö*pharmacognosy is the study of man's use of *animals* as medicines—bugs as drugs. Drugs of animal origin include serum vaccines, hormones, aphrodisiac beetles (spanish fly), immunostimulating ants, cod liver oil, deer musk, cat civet, psychoactive toad venoms, dream fish, and toxic honeys. These are things that people use. Animals also seek out drugs in their environment for medicinal use, such as purgative grasses. We have learned to observe these animal uses of healing plants for our own drug discovery, and indeed this may be how we humans developed most of our medicinal repertoire.

A further subdiscipline of ethnobotany is the study of psychoactive plant use, sometimes called *entheo*botany. Giorgio Samorini estimates that there are nearly 200 scientific researchers devoted to this emerging field of entheobotany, and among us, even fewer investigators of *entheozöö*pharmacognosy, or the use by humans of inebriating animal products. It follows that there is also a study of the use of *psychoactive* substances *by animals*. Yet there is currently no name for this line of study and— although it may be fun to create one—this lack of terminology is indicative of the appalling absence of scientific research in this area.

Animals do use drugs, and within this new study of animals medicating themselves exists the sphere that is the intriguing subject of this book: *animals intentionally inebriate themselves.* This book addresses the fact that animals drug themselves for more than medicinal purposes; they drug themselves for inebriation. Animals use drugs, and animals drug themselves.

As this book reveals, the occurrence of animals inebriating themselves is present throughout all levels of the animal world—present, but scattered. Within any species, inebriation-seeking behavior is not shared by all individuals. There may be a rather constant percentage of individuals—animals, birds, insects, and humans—for whom inebriation is a sought-after experience, an intentional impulse. It is not for everyone, so to speak, but there are positive indications that this special, altered minority contributes something beneficial for the ongoing development and adaptation of its species.

Could it be that animals that consume various plant inebriants develop enhanced senses and perceptual acuity that confer an adaptive advantage in evolution? Even strict biologists agree that behaviors leading to more successful food acquisition or hunting techniques increase survival. Suggestive evidence shows that altered states produced by certain psychoactive plants can allow rigid instincts to be bypassed, enabling new behaviors and techniques to be learned and passed along by the experimentalists of a species. Awareness-enhancing plant drugs are indeed sought out by certain animals. And behavior which increases mating, such as eating prosexual or libidostimulant plant drugs (the so-called aphrodisiacs), means disproportionate breeding by that savvy individual who thus breeds more of its gene type into the species.

Consider some of the latest discoveries in this ongoing study. Wild chimpanzees in the rainforests of tropical West Africa have been observed intentionally using medicinal plants, which these chimps seem to apply as effective antiparasitics. This chimp herbalist subculture must have developed long, long ago. Its documentation by Professor Michael Huffman of Kyoto University's Primate Research Institute is having tremendous impact on our understanding of these primates. Even more startling is Dr. Huffman's discovery of the recreational use of the drug plants for inebriation—*Alchornea floribunda* by gorillas and *A. cordifolia* by chimpanzees—as published in the journal African Studies Monographs, Winter 2002. *A. floribunda* is the source of the plant drug *alán,* a visionary intoxicant and aphrodisiac used by West African cults. Local people claim to have discovered these uses by observing gorillas become inebriated after eating the roots. The same is said by native Africans of the more widely known eboka, *Tabernanthe iboga,* a potent psychoactive root used in an initiation ceremony in the Bwiti religion in Gabon. Samorini himself is an initiate of this modern eboka order.

Gorillas really do know to dig roots of the iboga bush,

they know how to distinguish this particular species amongst the bewildering number of plants in the rainforest and selectively decide to eat these extremely bitter roots for the sole purpose of experiencing the impressive psychoactive effects produced by its indole alkaloids. One must remember that the task of finding such a nondescript rainforest bush in the wild is no simple matter. It requires a level of sophistication and learning thatmodern botanists rarely possess.

What can we conclude from the fact that there are ants engaged in an elaborate relationship with a species of beetle that they host in their nests? A *Coleopter* beetle whose inebriating abdominal secretions are so desired by the ants that, should the colony be disturbed, they forego rescuing their own larvae to protect the beetle, and even under nonemergency conditions the ants drug themselves to the point of losing their ability to work and creating sterile queens. Why do they do this?

Does it surprise us that reindeer eat fly agaric mushrooms or that bighorn sheep selectively seek out, and repeatedly consume, psychoactive lichen for the sake of an altered state of consciousness — not by accident, but with foreknowledge and premeditation?

Intention is at the crux of understanding the significance of these behaviors: whether the animals know what will happen from the drug experience and seek it out. Since these are indisputable facts, better we ask: Why would it surprise us? Is it that such behavior would be unique to humans, a kind of hallmark of intelligence or consciousness? Is knowledge and premeditation a precious defining line between animal and human consciousness? Why would we care to draw a line? In studying the drug-seeking behaviors of animals we may find answers that explain parallel human behavior. Do animals pursue psychoactive drugs for the same reasons as we humans do? If animals, birds, and, yes, even insects avail themselves of inebriation, then we must see this as a natural impulse to take drugs to alter consciousness, and it exists in man as well. Perhaps, then, the problem of "problem drugs" is no problem after all.

Fortunately science, and not soft thinking, surrounds the relevant disciplines relied upon as background in *Animals and Psychedelics*. Conclusions may be drawn, but they are always done so at the risk of being drawn *out*, attenuated by speculative deduction. Here is where Giorgio Samorini does not fail us. He thoroughly presents the most thought-provoking facts, arranging them for our contemplation without surrendering to conclusions. By bringing us to the vista point, showing us the expansive natural panorama, enumerating the many details, and presenting what is known about how it came to be, he leaves us to find our own *aha!*

ROB MONTGOMERY,
Founder of Botanical Preservation Corps

Introduction

DRUGS IN THE ANIMAL KINGDOM AND BEYOND

When we speak of drugs, most people immediately associate them with the "drug problem," bringing us to a communal vision that perceives drugs and the drug problem as identical. This negative connotation surrounding the concept of drugs is even more greatly exacerbated in a cultural environment that negates the slightest useful significance to the act of drugging oneself.

Drugs are harmful; drugs are a vice; drugs are symptoms of individual and social unease and suffering—such judgments, often implied, create in the collective mind the concept that the use of drugs is an aberrant behavior specific to the human species.

Contradicting this paradigm of modern Western thought is a collection of data that has become ever more conspicuous and incontestable—although it continues to be underestimated—that clearly demonstrates that self-drugging behavior is also widespread throughout the animal world. A few cases of animal addiction have been widely known for some time but not considered seriously, since researchers simply followed the rule—which Westerners vigorously obey—of not pursuing, not being interested in inexplicable data or facts in strong contradiction to established interpretive models. At best a scrupulous ethologist here or there interpreted these bizarre animal behaviors in psychological terms, as symptoms of some illness or imbalance in the animal, thus projecting onto the animal world the same pathological analysis attributed to the human species.

In the past few decades, however, with the adoption of ever more refined techniques of observation and the centralization of data gathered from every region of the globe, ethologists are accumulating a mass of factual information about animals that drug themselves voluntarily, so that the pertinent data can no longer be underestimated. What seemed at first to be an exception now appears to be, instead, a behavioral rule scattered throughout all levels of the animal world—from mammals to birds and even insects—so that the interpretation of such behavior as a particular and individualized symptom of illness is no longer valid and acceptable. One must suspect, instead, that in the behavior of animals—and therefore, of human beings—the consumption of drugs constitutes some natural component. In other words, the appropriate drug triggers, within a given animal, some natural function not yet understood. For a more in-depth analysis of the motivations that drive animals and humans to drug themselves, the reader can refer to the final chapter of this brief study.

The first references of a scientific character made to the use of drugs by animals seem to date back to the second half of the nineteenth century. Paolo Mantegazza, in his monumental work on drugs, reported that these "nerve nourishers," as he loved to define them, "are almost exclusively used by man, who is imbued with a nervous system and life more complex than all other animals. Among these, those who are closest to us in intelligence may find [drugs] pleasurable when they learn to know them in a condition of domestication. Monkeys, parrots, and even dogs often love coffee and tea to the point of transport; but in nature they do not know how to find them by instinct."

But in a footnote he was quick to add: "The progresses of science are greatly devaluing this last, too resolute statement. Perhaps not even the use of 'nerve nourishers' is a purely human characteristic: Cats eat catnip and valerian, surely not to feed themselves but to become intoxicated." So, too, Mrs. Loreau, Livingstone's trans- lator, states that elephants in some places search avidly for a certain fruit that inebriates them, enjoying their drunkenness very much. Darwin frequently observed monkeys, when given the opportunity, smoking with pleasure, and Brehm assures us that in northeastern Africa the natives capture monkeys by offering them pitchers full of a very strong beer that makes them drunk (Mantegazza 1871, 1:174–75).

Before going on to demonstrate the data on the various animals that drug themselves, I would like to pause and examine some of the definitions regarding the complex relationship of animals with drugs.

A primary problem concerns the very definition of what is or is not a drug. Such a definition is not precisely formulated in the field of human drugs and becomes even more problematic if we consider the drugs ingested by animals, since defining a given substance as a drug depends on the behavior that the use of the substance induces in a human being or animal.

If we think of drugging oneself in terms of dependence and addiction, we might define a drug as something that creates in its user a strong behavioral dependence, the deprivation of which brings on an obvious crisis of withdrawal. But then food, too, would conform to such a definition, since it is something on which we are continually dependent, the deprivation of which induces the most evident and critical withdrawal of all: hunger leading to potential starvation. Apart from this consideration, a substantial number of substances that human beings use as drugs do not induce any physical dependency, nor do they lead to crises of withdrawal—for example, the entire class of hallucinogens.

Or we could define drugs as those substances that act on the nervous system, but in this case, as well, the boundaries between drugs, medicines, and food are not clear. Various components in different foods and in the most commonly prescribed medicines affect the nervous system, and there are substances that act on the nervous system yet do not necessarily make the user feel drugged.

Furthermore, we could define drugs as any substances that, when ingested, lead to uncommon and bizarre behaviors. This would seemingly address the case of both people and elephants who drink alcohol. In fact, it is precisely the observation of bizarre behavior in animals following ingestion of a given substance that causes us to assume that the substance involved acts as a drug. But in this case, also, there are innumerable substances and types of behavior that escape such a pat definition. There are people, for example, who, after taking lysergic acid diethylamide (LSD), sit peacefully in an armchair — reading, writing, or simply thinking, without demonstrating any type of behavior that might lead a third party to believe them to be under the influence of a powerful hallucinogenic drug.

But then, what is it that makes a person say, "I feel drugged"? It is a mental dimension clearly recognizable as different from the person's ordinary mental dimension, induced by the administration of some determined substance that the individual and/or society in general characterizes as a drug. Yet even this is a limited definition. Most smokers do not even perceive the mental dimension induced by tobacco and consider themselves drugged only at the point in which they begin to recognize their addiction to cigarettes. (How many times I've heard people talk of "alcohol *and* drugs" or "tobacco *and* drugs," demonstrating their conviction, as erroneous as it is deep-seated, that alcohol and tobacco are not drugs, since they are not illegal substances!)

If we shift our attention to tribal populations, we find completely different definitions and concepts of what composes a drug. For example, according to various tribes native to Amazonia, drugs are those substances given to them by Westerners, such as alcohol and cigarettes. Meanwhile, the shamans of these tribes do not conceive of being addicted to the drugs they use traditionally— first among them being the local tobacco, called mapacho, which they smoke continually. For them this tobacco, along with a hallucinogenic drink called ayahuasca, are included in the category of medicines and nourishment of the soul.

From all this we can deduce that the definition of what constitutes a drug is dependent on its encompassing culture. Even the effects of drugs are influenced by the cultural environment in which they are experienced. For this reason it is extremely difficult to formulate a scientific and general definition of the concepts *drug* and *drugged*. It is also probable that some of these difficulties are reinforced by excessive generalization regarding the drug phenomenon; that is to say, many behavioral phenomena are forced together under this umbrella concept, when in reality they are sharply distinct from it. What a long road we have yet to walk before reaching an objective and scientific analysis of the drug phenomenon!

Shifting our attention yet again to observe the animal world, the situation becomes, understandably, even more complicated, given that animals cannot communicate their sensation of feeling drugged to us, and we must therefore deduce their condition through observation of their outward behavior or, at best, by physiological and neuropharmacological data. Considering that our concept of what it means to be drugged is culturally biased, observation of drugged animals runs the serious risk of being nonobjective. Scientific research—not excluding ethology—generally follows the principle of "finding what you're looking for," and both research and researchers are conditioned by a cultural and moral environment that dictates a priori that in human behavior, the use of drugs is an aberrant phenomenon completely lacking in constructive value. We should not be surprised, therefore, if the study of such behavior among animals is still in its first stages. In the nonpermissive cultural matrix that surrounds us, it is difficult to affirm and accept that the "filthy" habit of drugging oneself could corrupt the "purity" of animal nature. For an ethologist to make such a statement is tantamount to sending his professional career up in smoke.

A second class of problems regards the *intention* of the animal in the act of drugging itself. We must, from the start, distinguish the behavior of animals that drug themselves because they are influenced or directly induced by human beings to do so from the behavior of animals in the wild that choose to drug themselves without any apparent human influence.

In the opium dens of the Orient, domestic cats become

addicted to the opium smoke permeating the rooms, and it is common to see these cats approach the smokers, waiting for them to expel mouthfuls of smoke, which the animals then inhale repeatedly. That these creatures are addicted to opium is proved by the fact that normal cats turn away in disgust to avoid the exhaled smoke, as well as the fact that when the opium-den cats are deprived of their daily fumes, they are seized by obvious symptoms of withdrawal, which in some cases result in their death. Even the mice that live in and around the dens approach the smokers—who are generally undisturbed by the intrusion—and stand up on their hind legs in an attempt to inhale the opium.

In Africa, monkeys who live in captivity and in direct contact with cigarette smokers swiftly take up the habit of smoking themselves and become infuriated if they are denied their daily cigarettes. I witnessed this myself during the course of my field studies in Gabon. In such cases we are clearly not dealing with a natural animal impulse but with an intentional behavior conditioned by the human environment in which these animals live.

Nor can we consider it a natural impulse in those cases in which human beings themselves are the ones to administer by force certain drugs to laboratory animals for the purposes of research. Journals specializing in psychopharmacological and neurochemical research are filled with the results of experiments carried out on the most disparate animals, who undergo forced administration of cocaine, heroin, nicotine, and countless other drugs so that scientists can study their physical and behavioral effects. In certain cases the animals in question are trained to self-administer the drugs, for the purpose of researching the mechanisms and parameters of addiction, tolerance, and crises of withdrawal, as well as the subjects' instincts, emotions, and social relationships under the effect of whatever drug is being studied. Such cases are not relevant to our interests here, either, in that they constitute intentionally forced behavior dictated by human will.

This particular research, then, focuses solely on those cases in which animals evidence a natural intentional behavior in their consumption of drugs, far removed from any human influence.

Having verified the absolute impossibility of human influence, we must next distinguish between accidental and intentional ingestion, a distinction not always immediately evident. Ethologists frequently tend to interpret cases of animals that become intoxicated by consuming psychoactive plants as accidental. But our knowledge of incontestable cases in which ingestion was *not* accidental should give rise to doubt as to whether, hidden behind the theory of chance mishap usually attributed by broader surveys to the relationship between animals and psychoactive drugs, there might not simply lie our ignorance of both intimate and generalized behaviors in the animal world.

The interpretation of accidental ingestion is justified to a certain extent in that the behavior of animals that drug themselves brings with it, in many cases, a certain risk in apparent contradiction to the instinct for self-preservation. Moths that grow drunk on the nectar of the datura flower fall to the ground in a daze and remain there for some time, running the risk of being swallowed by predators; Canadian caribou, after intoxicating themselves by eating fly-agaric mushrooms, wander away from their calves, which then become frequent victims of wolves; American robins that gobble down certain kinds of berries and get drunk fall to the ground and are often run over by cars or eaten by cats. Although such dire costs contradict the individual instinct of self-preservation, it does not follow that they are contradictory if we observe the phenomenon in terms of the species.

One criterion for distinguishing between accidental and intentional behaviors is whether or not such behaviors are engaged in repeatedly. If we observe a goat eat the inebriant beans of the mescal plant and afterward tremble, fall down, and rise up again later, we might well consider the goat to have undergone an accidental intoxication by a psychoactive drug. But when we observe the same goat

11

return time and again to eat those same beans, manifesting identical symptoms of inebriation each and every time, it must make us suspect an intentional behavior of which the outward symptoms—trembling, falling to the earth, and getting back up in a while—are only some of the effects, probably the least important ones, of the drunkenness that goat is experiencing, to which it is attracted in some way and in which it is probably taking a certain pleasure. Shaking followed by lying down and then standing up again after a certain period of time is something that happens to many human beings who have consumed drugs of various types; yet we cannot, for this reason, affirm that the most significant effect of those drugs is that of shaking, falling down, and getting up again.

What types of drugs do animals use? The little we know at this point indicates that they are essentially vegetable in nature: seeds, the nectar of flowers, leaves, roots, fermented fruits, lichens, mushrooms, and so forth. In other words, plants. In most cases the drugs contained in plants that exert an intoxicating effect on human beings do the same for animals, but among the drugs used intentionally by animals, not all are used as drugs by people. Either their effect on humans is simply not known, or they have proven to be toxic to us. The mind-altering properties of many drugs found in plants—coffee, tea, khat, iboga, and fly agaric, for instance—were discovered by human observers who initially witnessed their intentional use by animals.

That drugs affecting human beings also affect animals has been proved by countless experiments in which these same drugs were administered to the most disparate animal species. Even the so-called inferior animals undergo similar effects. Still famous are the experiments carried out on spiders to whom appropriate doses of different drugs were orally administered. Every once in a while a meal of flies containing these drugs was fed to spiders of the genus *Zilla x notata,* which were then observed building their webs while in a mind-altered state. Under the influence of LSD the webs were characteristically arabesque, while caffeine-affected webs appeared angular, with sharp corners and large empty spaces that rendered them useless; under the influence of hashish, the webs were functional, but they were only partially filled in. (Stafford 1979).

In another experiment, different doses of LSD were administered orally to some hornets *(Vespa orientalis).* About ten minutes after the ingestion of this powerful hallucinogen, the insects manifested a slowing down of their movements, then the cessation of all activity, stereotypical motions, and states of apparent lethargy (Floru, Ishay, and Gitter 1969). These behavioral changes, while revealing nothing to us of the inner sensations experienced by the hornets, demonstrate that

LSD does, incontrovertibly, affect the hymenopterans in question.

Other experiments still famous today are those that John Lilly undertook with dolphins into whom he injected LSD. It is well known that these cetaceans are highly intelligent and graced with a complex system of communication made up of whistles and vocalizations.

"If we put a second dolphin in with the first, who has been injected with LSD, the index of vocalization rises for a period of three hours; in other words, a real and true communicative exchange takes place. The other [noninjected] dolphin responds to the first, and his index of vocalization augments as well. If a person enters the tank while [the dolphin is under] the effect of LSD, the vocalization index rises and remains high. Without LSD it rises for only a brief period of time."

That LSD evokes a socializing effect on dolphins was also demonstrated by an experiment conducted with a male dolphin who had rebuffed all contact with human beings for two and a half years after having been accidentally struck in the tail by an underwater speargun. Under the influence of LSD, the dolphin approached Lilly and his collaborators for the first time and remained near them for the entire period of affect by the hallucinogen (Lilly 1981, 240).

Even among animals whose diet is exclusively

carnivorous, we know of cases in which they have sought out and ingested vegetable material, sometimes—but not always—for the purpose of self-intoxication. There are some known cases of animals that use plants as medicines, and such behavior is probably much more widespread than we know of as yet.

Cats are wont to chew the young leaves and blades of certain grasses as emetics to purge their digestive systems. Chimpanzees of the species *Pan troglodytes*, who live in Tanzania, use the leaves of a species of *Aspilia*, belonging to the Asteraceae family, for medicinal purposes. These leaves contain thiarubrine-A, a powerful antibacterial and antifungal agent, and are traditionally used for medicinal reasons by the human populations of Tanzania (Rodriguez et al. 1985). The chimpanzees gather these leaves "usually first thing in the morning. The leaves are not chewed but held in the mouth and massaged against the gums with the tongue. It has been hypothesized that this technique evolved among the chimps to augment absorption of the active principle administered by mouth, since the moment it enters the acid environment of the stomach it becomes deactivated. We use similar methods for the consumption of pharmaceuticals sensitive to gastric juices. . . . We have even witnessed an anorexic and obviously sick chimpanzee lick the bitter juices from the pith of a particular tree *(Vernonia amygdalina)*. Presumably the afflicted animal had actively sought out the plant, despite its unpleasant taste, precisely for its medicinal virtues (McGowan 1999, 331; Newton and Nishida 1991)."

Baboons of the genus *Papio* eat the fruit of *Balanites aegyptica*, probably not as food but for its curative properties, given that it contains elevated quantities of dioxin, a steroid efficient in countering the larval stages of trematodes, a kind of parasitic flatworm (McGowan 1999, 332).

Perhaps one day we'll know much more about animals that cure themselves, just as we'll know more about animals that drug themselves. The boundary between medicine and drug has never been clear in the human world — as demonstrated by the fact that all drugs are also powerful medicines — and almost certainly the same holds true for the animal kingdom.

In the following chapters I will recount in detail the data gathered thus far on animals that drug themselves, basing my reports, essentially, on scientific writings on the subject. I am aware that these data are not exhaustive and that my work suffers somewhat in its system of bibliographic referencing. This is because what I am trying to draw attention to here — *natural and intentional behavior* interpretable as drug use in the animal world — is something that is, even now, underestimated, for the most part accorded little value or at the least interpreted in some other way.

What follows, then, represents the first collection of
data on the subject in its entirety, a first step toward the
acceptance of something that is still considered largely
inadmissible. All this simply follows the normal process
of acceptance of any new idea: initially derided and
opposed, it eventually forces an opening, or point of
passage, through which rigid modes of thought and
preestablished interpretive models can disintegrate. The
new idea then flows forward until it attains complete
acceptance and becomes incorporated into the common
baggage of human cognitive experience.

I would have made little headway in my research
without Ronald K. Siegel's brilliant text *Intoxication: Life
in Pursuit of Artificial Paradise,* published in the United
States in 1989. Siegel has conducted research and
observations of animals ingesting drugs both in the field
and in the laboratory; in his book he has gathered a dense
body of documentation on the subject, which I have
referred to again and again in the course of my own work.

1

CRAZED COWS

One of the most well known and striking examples of addictive behavior—that is, of true drug addiction—in animals involves locoweed, also called crazy grass or crazy seeds. This is a dense group of different kinds of wild grasses (at least forty) that spring up weedlike in the fields and belong, for the most part, to the legume family and are psychoactive for a variety of animals. So far, the animals we know to be affected by addiction to locoweed (a condition known as locoism) include mules, donkeys, horses, cows, sheep, antelopes, pigs, rabbits, and hens.

The most sensational cases of locoism by far have been reported in North America. As far as we know, this behavior was first described in 1873 in California, as a result of observing the actions of horses and cows browsing at pasture. The most curious aspect of their behavior was that once an animal had learned to differentiate the specific grass that brought on intoxication from the numerous other kinds of grass it ingested, it would habitually seek out and consume that particular plant. Foals, calves, and other offspring of mothers who eat crazy grass are likewise addicted and soon learn to distinguish and seek out the intoxicating plant.

Farmers in Kansas will never forget the terrible tales of the crazy grass epidemic of 1883, during which twenty-five thousand cows ceased eating normal pasture grasses almost completely, devoting themselves instead to an obstinate search for locoweed, less nourishing but — for some reason — more enticing. In 1938 Reko, working in Nebraska, identified *Astragalus lambertii* as locoweed, while in the vast prairies between Mexico and Montana, and reaching all the way into central Arizona, it was the dense and diffuse *Astragalus mollissimus* that earned the same rubric. A third species scattered throughout the prairies and meadowlands was *Cystium diphysum* (Reko 1996, 186–89). And a fourth locoweed was identified as *Dioon edule*, from the single surviving family of Cycadaceae, a palmlike tropical plant.

There is yet another crazy grass, which Mexicans call *garbancillo (Astragalus amphyoxis)*. Animals who have consumed it isolate themselves from the others, avoiding all companionship. They eat almost nothing, lose weight rapidly, and become extremely ill-tempered. If an attempt is made to lead them back to the herd, they rigidify and refuse to move. After balking completely, they distance themselves even farther from the flock.

In some cases, such animals are gripped by states of intense agitation and fury. Without any apparent reason, they may hurl themselves, bellowing and snorting, at other animals or human beings, even those with whom they have enjoyed daily contact. Within a brief period of time the symptoms of abnormality multiply. The creatures begin to walk with an uncertain, heavy, stumbling gait, hind parts swaying; quite often they come to a halt, their legs splayed wide as if to better support them and stare fixedly to the front with bulging eyes. Every once in a while they are seized by a convulsed shuddering. These conditions share a remarkable affinity with the so-called symptoms of withdrawal manifested by alcoholics, especially during certain stages of detoxification. Also striking is the fact that the affected animals, dazed as they are, seem not to recognize obstacles; they trip frequently, smacking their heads against tree trunks or telephone poles and fail to move aside for other animals.

However, the moment they are able to escape from the herd and browse on their beloved forage, they are swiftly renewed, becoming vivacious, vigorous, and energetic—even exuberant. Suddenly nothing in their behavior suggests any illness at all. Sometimes the reaction is different, however: an addicted animal may be found hiding somewhere, behind boulders or among the trees, in a state of profound prostration, either sitting up with its head erect and immobile or lying on the ground, its nose pointed upward and its eyes fixed and bulging, in a condition we can only describe as advanced drunkenness. Every so often it is seized by muscular cramps; also noticeable are a peculiar quivering of the eyelids and a squinty, cross-eyed stare directed at the sky. And as in all cases of poisoning, the animal's breathing undergoes strange alterations, often becoming a labored panting. The breathing of healthy cows is characterized by deep inhalations followed by long pauses, but animals intoxicated by locoweed breathe brokenly, in quick, strained inhalations and brief exhalations, followed by short pauses.

Chachaquila (Oxytropis lambertii), another type of locoweed especially enticing to bovids, produces a peculiar kind of intoxication accompanied by hallucinations and high excitement. Animals already familiar with the plant will suddenly hurl themselves free of the herd and escape, as if seized by the Furies, toward the very places herders most assiduously avoid: sites where the chachaquila grows. Following these berserk beasts is not only futile but inadvisable, since in their condition of withdrawal and craving they are fully capable of throwing themselves off cliffs or running from their pursuers at such wild speeds that they can drop dead of heart attacks. If the animals can be kept away from the dangerous grasses and held under scrupulous attention so that they do not wander off from the herd, their symptoms of excitation and withdrawal apparently diminish without further consequence and their psychic equilibrium reestablishes itself. This in itself, however, is not enough to cure them of the addiction. If rehabilitated cows later stumble upon their drug of choice they take up where they left off—eating it avidly, becoming deeply intoxicated, and, in the digestive phase that follows, irritable and aggressive (Reko 1996, 186–89).

A surprising fact is that the more interested the browsing animals become in locoweed, the more widely it springs up in the pasture, becoming after a while the dominant plant.

Many pastures have had to be abandoned by cattle farmers altogether, having been so invaded by locoweed that no other grasses can grow there. This may be caused by the scattering of seeds in the animals' droppings or by some other, as yet unknown, ecological factor.

Despite the repressive measures adopted by farmers (attempted eradication of the crazy grass, separation of newborn calves, foals, and lambs from their addicted mothers, and so on), the tenacity of the plant itself and of the animals in seeking it out and ingesting it remains one of the most ruinous scourges of North American zootechnics.

One characteristic of locoism is precisely that tenacity—the stubbornness with which addicted animals seek out the inebriant plant. Even as farmers were eradicating the locoweed from certain pastures, for instance, cows and horses were observed stealing the sacks in which the grass had been gathered, even overturning the wagons in which the sacks had been packed. Horses in the grip of hallucinations and uncontrollable attacks of mania after having devoured the flowers and leaves of locoweed dig into the earth with their hooves to extract and eat the roots.

Unfortunately, many addicted animals die even before the intrinsic toxicity of the locoweed can kill them, succumbing to malnourishment and starvation, since, in their single-minded search for the drug—which becomes, at last, their sole focus in life — they cease to eat other, more nourishing grasses. In the United States there are actual retreats dedicated to the recovery of animals addicted to locoweed, in which an attempt is made to rehabilitate them, interrupting the cycle of dependency so that they can be reintroduced to their proper work — that is, nourishing themselves healthily so as to attain a desirable weight, to be directed toward their more "natural" end: slaughter. Before long, perhaps, American supermarket shoppers will be able to purchase, at competitive prices, the meat of recovered cows, horses, and pigs!

The widespread problem of locoweed madness in cattle is probably a consequence of intensive breeding and raising, and so indirectly influenced by human practices. In other words, the frenzied drug use we observe in these animals may be due to their massively crowded condition, dictated by human exigency. Since cows do not exist in the wild, we have been unable to observe the phenomenon as it might occur in a natural state. Unless we discover other grazing quadrupeds free of human interference seeking out and eating locoweed, the question will remain open.

Various types of locoweed are toxic — generally neurotoxic — to human beings, while others, taken as teas, induce tranquilization and a mild sensation of detachment from the surrounding world. Higher doses result in overstimulation and hallucinations (Siegel, 1989, 52–54).

Loco intoxication is not confined to North America but is found to a greater or lesser degree on every continent. In Australia, grazing animals attracted by the leguminous *Swainsonia galegifolia* are called indigo eaters; like North American cows, they isolate themselves from the herd, suffer hallucinations, and feed on the drug to the exclusion of all other grasses. In Europe one of the most common locoweeds is broom *(Cytisus scoparius)*, also a leguminous plant capable of producing psychoactive or toxic effects in human beings, according to the dose. When given in low doses to sheep, however, the plant encourages vivacious behavior. L. Lewin, in his *Phantastika,* reports that "certain breeds of sheep native to the German moors are partial to it. It is therefore frequently planted on the heathlands, and the sheep are herded slowly across them without being given a chance to halt. Certain animals eat it greedily and passionately and so enter a state of excitation followed by complete loss of consciousness. Such creatures easily fall prey to foxes or flocks of crows. They are known as 'the drunkards.'" (Lewin 1981, 2: 179.)

Different types of crazy grass belong to the legume family and to the *Astragalus, Oxytropis,* and *Lathyrus* genera. The active principle miserotoxin, poisonous to humans, has been identified in the first two, while neurolathyritic compounds are present in the third. These neruolathyrogens, aside from inducing advanced drunkenness in animals, also effect a state of toxicity in humans. This state, known as neurolathyrogenic, was epidemic in the past during times of famine when flour for bread making was cut with the seeds and pods of *Lathyrus*, popularly known as vetch or tare (Camporesi 1980). Lathyrism is characterized, among other things, by spastic paralysis in the lower limbs of human beings and the hind limbs of domestic animals.

Other species of locoweed in America are *Croton fruticulosus* (Euphorbiaceae), *Lobelia cliffordiana* (Lobeliaceae), and *Lupinus elegans* (Leguminosae).

Studies of the Australian locoweed *Swainsonia canescens* have revealed the presence of the alkaloid indolizine, responsible for loco intoxication in animals. This same indolizine alkaloid, as well as its by-product N-oxide, is also present in *Astragalus lentiginosus*, the spotted locoweed found in Utah (Molyneux and James 1982).

2

aLCOHOL AND ANIMALS: from DRUNKEN eLePHANTS to SAUCED SNAILS

Pachyderms' passion for alcohol has long been famous. African elephants are avid for the fruits of several kinds of palm tree: doum, marula, mgongo, and palmyra *(Borassus)*. As they ripen, these fruits tend to ferment swiftly, sometimes while still attached to the tree. Elephants will devour the fermented fruits already scattered over the earth and then shake the tree, beating it with their trunks and bodies until further fruits fall. Fermentation of these fruits produces ethyl alcohol in concentrations as high as 7 percent, and this process continues when the fruit enters the animals' digestive systems, resulting in the production and absorption of even greater quantities of alcohol. To compound matters, groups of elephants appear to compete over the fruits, each of them trying to eat the most fruit in the shortest time possible. Their consequent drunkenness is anything but accidental; they are quite clearly *seeking* a state of intoxication. Although a herd usually ranges no more than about six miles through the forest on a given day, when these palm fruits (especially those of the *Borassus*) ripen, adult males may distance themselves from the herd and cover more than twenty miles in a day to reach trees whose location they retain firmly in their memories.

Once drunk, the elephants become overexcited and tend to jump and startle at unusual sounds or sudden movements on the part of other animals or human beings. They scare easily and react defensively, becoming extremely aggressive. A herd of drunken elephants is considered a serious danger to humans.

Elephants live in structured groups with matriarchal hierarchies. A young elephant will commonly put its trunk inside its mother's mouth to take and taste what she is eating, thus learning what to choose for itself. If its mother is feeding on fermenting fruit, her calf will become intoxicated as well, learning early on to appreciate and seek out a state of inebriation.

"This information is retained and used when a female calf grows up and becomes the new matriarch. Then younger animals learn from her, and a local tradition is established. The collective wisdom of centuries can be carried by these animals unless a matriarch is killed by poachers and the chain is broken. Thus the seasonal binges on alcohol become part of elephant behavior (Siegel 1989, 119–20)."

The Asian elephants of Bengal and Indonesia are also attracted to fallen fermented fruits, especially the enormous, heavy fruits of the durian, or *Durio zibethinus*. Actually, many different kinds of animals eagerly seek out fermented durian fruit: monkeys, orangutans, honey bears, squirrels, flying foxes (fruit bats), elephants, and human beings. Even Sumatran tigers, the ultimate carnivores, make an exception for durian, although it is not clear whether they appreciate it for its intoxicating effect or eat it for some other reason. But their passionate determination to possess it is well known among the native people of Sumatra, who report cases in which children carrying baskets of durian back to their villages were attacked by tigers, which, instead of killing them, simply stole their harvest.

Elephants that have feasted on durian tend to sway and fall down, lolling on the earth in a state of lethargy. Monkeys lose motor coordination, roll their heads, and climb trees only with great effort. Flying foxes, the largest bats in the world, feed on fermented durian fruits in the night. Their ensuing intoxication distorts the complex radar system by which they orient themselves during their nocturnal flights to such a degree that they frequently fall to the ground.

Elephants do not limit their search for a high to fermented fruits alone but rapidly head in the direction of any source emanating the scent of alcohol. In western Bengal in 1985 a herd of 150 elephants burst into a clandestine laboratory and gulped down an enormous quantity of distilled malt liquor. Wildly drunk, they roved around the nearby territory, galloping in all directions and crushing and killing five people. A dozen or so other people were injured and seven brick homes and about twenty huts were destroyed. Dumbo, the imaginary flying elephant of cartoon fame who sees dancing pink elephants himself after drinking alcohol, originated from the knowledge of his real, wild prototypes' fondness for drink.

Fruits and other vegetation subject to fermentation inebriate various species of animals — not only mammals but birds and even insects. In the American West, for example, sapsuckers — a kind of woodpecker — use their beaks to drill holes in trees to feed on the sap that oozes into them. Exposed to the proper temperature, this sap will ferment, producing alcohol. It then attracts various other animals, such as hummingbirds, squirrels, and other woodpeckers, who get drunk while feeding on the fermented sap in the pit created by the first bird. Most such cases are considered to be inadvertent—accidental ingestions of alcohol in the guise of nourishment. But given the tendency on the part of scholarly researchers to negate any natural elements in animal drug use, we cannot be too certain of this.

It seems that even slugs and snails are attracted to alcohol. Farmers and gardeners in Italy and elsewhere make use of this fact to rid orchards or gardens of both by putting out low, wide containers (plastic flowerpot saucers are perfect) into which they have poured a little beer or wine. The mollusks are easily enticed into such traps, converging on them in the dozens from every direction, piling up one on top of another. The heaps of slugs or snails, apparently drunk and unable to move, can then be simply scooped up and eliminated.

Farmers in northern Italy have long used a similar method to invite hedgehogs to live in their gardens. Hedgehogs are formidable insectivores, and their presence in any garden guarantees that cabbages and salad greens will flourish undevoured by the bugs. Since these little mammals are also partial to alcohol, placing a bowl of watered wine with a handful of slugs in the middle of the garden every so often is a surefire way to ensure that they'll settle down there (Celli 1999, 15–16).

3
fRenzied feLines

Many members of the feline
family, from domestic cats to
tigers, become intoxicated after
eating or chewing the leaves of
certain herbs. The most well
known example, of course, is the
behavior of cats around *Nepeta
cataria,* or catnip. *Nepeta* grows
wild in uncultivated fields, and
the dried leaves are commercially
available as well, usually sewn
into little bags or pillows and

sold as "rejuvenating and invigorating" toys for domestic cats. *Nepeta* should not be confused with another cat herb sold in pet stores, which is a type of grass whose stems, when chewed, induce vomiting in cats and act to purge their digestive systems.

When a cat is offered catnip, its behavior is observable as a succession of four separate stages. First the cat sniffs the plant (which smells like mint and/or alfalfa to humans); second, it licks the leaves and sometimes chews them. Ronald K. Siegel says in *Intoxication: Life in Pursuit of Artificial Paradise* that the "chewing is often interrupted when the cat momentarily stares into space with a blank expression, then quickly shakes its head from side to side. In the third stage the cat will usually rub against the plant with its chin and cheek. Last, there is a 'head over' roll with rubbing of the entire body. Extremely sensitive cats may also flip from side to side by rolling over on their backs. The four-stage reaction runs its fixed course in approximately ten minutes. . . . The nature of the pleasurable intoxication becomes increasingly evident when high doses of catnip in the form of concentrated extracts are offered to the animals. The subsequent reactions are intense: cats head-twitch violently, salivate profusely, and show other signs of central nervous system excitation. Males have spontaneous erections, while females adopt mating stances, complete with vocalization and 'love-biting' of any available object.

"The similarity of the catnip response to the normal sexual behavior of cats is striking. The presentation of catnip results in the rolling pattern of behavior that is exhibited by estrus females during the course of normal sexual displays. These displays have prompted naturalists to speculate that catnip once served the evolutionary function in the wild of preparing cats for sex, a natural springtime aphrodisiac" (Siegel 1989, 62–63).

But domestic cats, many of whom pass their entire lives without ever seeing a catnip plant, are losing the capacity to feel the effect of *their* drug; current studies show that only 50 to 70 percent of indoor cats respond to catnip at all. Research has shown that the response or lack of response to the plant by a given cat is determined by the presence or absence of a particular gene. Perpetuation of generation after generation of cats raised without contact with catnip is genetically impoverishing these animals by depriving them of the possibility of response to their own natural drug (Todd 1962).

Other studies, conducted by G. F. Palen and G. V. Goddard in 1966, have yielded the following observations: "A typical 'body rolling' begins with the cat pressing his face to the floor and rubbing his jaw back and forth, progressively lengthening his body with paws outstretched before him, ears tipped forward, and claws out. The cat then rolls his head and entire body from one side to another. The duration of this rolling is extremely variable, lasting from a few seconds to four or five minutes, and is repeated from one to fifteen times. This reaction to catnip occurs independently of sex or age."

Responsive cats given the opportunity of contact with catnip seek it out daily. Specific ethological studies have demonstrated that these cats are as "happy" and healthy as cats who have no contact with the drug, if not more so. I can personally vouch for the frequency of this habit as seen in the cats that come daily to visit the catnip plant growing in my garden. My garden is frequented by all the cats in the neighborhood, especially in springtime, when they come into heat and the plant is at the height of its vegetative phase, generously filling the air with its mentholated perfume. Toward the end of spring, when the plant flowers, its scent diminishes — as do the visits of the cats to my garden. My catnip plant seems to be the only one in the area, and at certain times in the spring, especially in late afternoon, my garden is crawling with cats. They don't seem to enjoy sharing their experiences with the plant but instead maintain a certain distance from each other: each cat waits for its own turn when the area around the catnip is free of undesired colleagues. Males and females approach it indiscriminately.

Nepeta cataria, like many of its congenerous species, produces volatile terpenoids called nepetalactones. These are the compounds responsible for the plant's intoxicating effect on felines, from domestic cats to tigers. They exert a psychoactive effect on human beings as well, although it is very slight. Laboratory research has shown that catnip also intoxicates other animal species, from insects to mice, modifying their behavior markedly. Nepetalic acid is the most potent of the various compounds produced by this plant (Harney, Leary, and Barofsky 1974).

Pheromones similar in structure to nepetalactones are present in the urine of male cats. This may well be why cats respond to catnip with behavior that is sexual in nature. But cats drugged on *Nepeta cataria* also seem to experience actual hallucinations. They have been observed grabbing at nonexistent things, playing with phantom butterflies apparently fluttering about them in the air, and lowering their ears to pounce on invisible mice. Some become fearful and defensive, hissing at nonexistent threats.

Another herb that exerts a psychoactive effect on cats is common valerian, a medicinal plant utilized by humans since antiquity as a sedative, antispasmodic, and mild narcotic. By the 1800s we find references to it as an herb for cats as well. The Neapolitan doctor Raffaele Valieri, for example, reported that "when a sack of valerian is scattered on the earth, it is a curious and enjoyable spectacle to watch cats approach it: they roll on top of it, inhale it repeatedly, and finally begin to tremble, their fur standing on end, then leap about disjointedly, making a thousand dancing gestures of unbridled, drunken bliss, and finally losing their senses and falling into a doze, remaining excited and dazed for a long time. And this is an analogous phenomenon, similar to the trembling, intoxication, phantasmagoria, and stupefaction that hashish induces in man" (Valieri 1887, 16).

Japanese cats enjoy a different drug, the tender leaves of a plant called matatabi, which produces compounds similar to nepetalactones. Matatabi exerts a wholly different effect than catnip on the creatures: after chewing its leaves, they stretch out on their backs with their paws up and remain motionless in this position for some time, in apparent or perhaps real ecstasy.

Offering your own beloved cats a cat herb means giving them the chance for a relationship with their own particular ancestral plant, allowing them to intoxicate themselves at their own whim with a natural and healthy drug without any danger of chronic addiction. The rapport cats enjoy with catnip, valerian, and related plants is a naturally seasonal one, particularly heightened in the spring; they are not subject to crises of withdrawal during the lengthy periods of the year when the plants lose their efficacy as inebriants. We do so much—at times the most absurd things—to procure happiness for ourselves. Yet so little suffices—a small plant on the windowsill of an urban apartment—to bring joy to our feline friends.

4

MUSHROOM-LOVING REINDEER AND CRAVING CARIBOU

A long-famous case of animals addicted to the use of a psychoactive drug is that of Siberian reindeer, who feed on the hallucinogenic fungus *Amanita muscaria*, or fly agaric. This is *the* hallucinogenic mushroom par excellence, the beautiful mushroom of fairy tales whose bright red cap is sprinkled with white spots. The origins of its use as a hallucinogen by human beings is lost in the dawn of time; archeological and ethnographic data have confirmed the early spread of this practice through- out Asia, Europe, and the Americas (Samorini 2001).

Fly agaric grows under certain types of trees, particularly conifers and birches. During the Siberian summer, the reindeer feed on a variety of mushrooms, among other things, but their favorite by far is the fly agaric found in birch forests. They hunt specifically for this showy fungus, seeking it out for the inebriation it provides them. After they have eaten it they run around aimlessly, make strange noises, twitch their heads, and isolate themselves from the rest of the herd. The tiniest bite of fly agaric induces in these reindeer a marked condition of intoxication characterized, above all, by continual head twitching, one of the most widespread manifestations of inebriation in all animals.

It is well known that the urine of humans who have eaten fly agaric becomes in itself hallucinogenic. Among some Siberian populations it was customary to drink the urine of those who had drugged themselves with the mushroom to attain an even greater degree of intoxication, reputedly more powerful than that achieved by eating the mushroom itself. Even reindeer "go mad" for the urine of other reindeer or human beings who have ingested the hallucinogen. In fact, it would seem that the Siberian peoples discovered its inebriating properties by observing the behavior of the reindeer. Anytime these creatures scent fungus-rich urine in the vicinity, they make a mad dash for it, engaging in real battles among themselves as they vie for the positions closest to the "golden shower."

Squirrels and chipmunks seek out fly agaric as well, nibbling at it and becoming intoxicated. This is probably also true, as we shall see later, of ordinary flies.

Other great seekers of the mushroom high are Canadian caribou. During their migrations these animals move in a long, single-file column. When the colony passes a cluster of *Amanita muscaria*, female adults feed on it greedily. Within the course of one or two hours, they abandon the column entirely, running about awkwardly and shaking their heads and hindquarters from side to side. Such behavior carries a certain cost for the herd as a whole, since mothers in their hallucinatory seizures temporarily abandon their young, leaving them unprotected, so that they often fall victim to wolves. Even the adult caribou, once isolated from their peers and made ungainly by their drugged condition, become frequent prey to the waiting wolves (Siegel 1989, 66–67).

A variety of animals feed on diverse psilocybin mushrooms, most commonly on *Psilocybe* and *Panaeolus*, which are popularly known as *funghetti* by young Italians who seek them out for their hallucinogenic effects (Pagani 1993).

Siegel relates having seen dogs in Hawaii and Mexico deliberately nipping the caps off psilocybin mushrooms and swallowing them. After only a few minutes the creatures were running in circles, shaking their heads, howling and barking, and refusing to obey human commands (Siegel 1989, 68). Although it is unclear whether the dogs were conscious of what would happen to them after ingestion of the mushrooms, there is no such question about intentionality in the case of goats. These peculiar ruminants seem to enjoy absolute supremacy in the animal world as far as their passion for disparate drugs is concerned.

In the course of my field research on the hallucinogenic mushrooms growing in Italy's alpine meadows (Samorini 1993), I have personally observed on several occasions the greed with which goats will devour the species *Psilocybe semilanceata*. Once I was actually assaulted by a large billy goat, which gave me a shove with his powerful horns while I was bent over to observe some funghetti. He was one of the more massive animals in a herd of about fifty that was rambling by me. Trusting in their harmlessness (though aware of their curiosity), I simply continued gathering the mushrooms. When I saw that several goats had stopped to watch me, I smiled at them ingenuously and showed them the bunch of mushrooms I had just harvested. The moment I did so, the buck leaped forward and shoved me sharply with his horns, causing me to roll several feet down the slope. During my tumble the paper bag holding the mushrooms I had collected fell out of my hand. Surprised and frightened, I remained at a distance from the buck, who, with several other goats, threw himself on the sack and devoured its contents. When it was empty, the animals began rooting through the grass, gobbling up all the mushrooms I had not yet collected.

Ever since, when I've encountered a bunch of goats, I've followed the advice of a knowledgeable goatherd and brandished my stick on high; it is the only way to stop them. And when I stumble onto a psilocybin site already claimed by goats, I make no attempt to drive them off— partly out of respect for them, but partly from fear of being attacked by animals already under the influence of this powerful drug and therefore doubly recalcitrant and dangerous.

Once they locate a cluster of psilocybin mushrooms, goats will not eat grass or any other kind of fungus, feeding exclusively on their drug of choice. It seems clear that they know how to recognize it and that they search it out for its psychoactive effects. Goats under its influence exhibit overstimulated behavior, run about awkwardly, and shake their heads wildly back and forth.

5

GALLOPING GOATS

There is a widespread tale in Ethiopia regarding the origin of coffee, which credits the discovery of its stimulating properties to a goatherd who happened to notice the bizarre behavior of his goats after they had browsed on coffee berries.

"Kaldi knew that something was wrong with the goats. During the hot days on the Ethiopian highlands they leaped around

43

the rocks, climbing impossible slopes, then descending in controlled slides and falls. At sunset they usually slept, lying with outstretched limbs, motionless as the mountain itself. Tonight they gamboled uncontrollably, bleating and chasing one another as their eyes darted in all directions. ... Kaldi noticed that the goats paused only to nibble the red berries from a nearby shrub, then continued to prance in the moonlight. The goats often behaved in unexpected ways, hence their flighty or capricious reputation, but Kaldi had never seen them approach this plant. He knew that the goats always test their food by scent and taste and prefer familiar foods. They especially like leaves; but strange berries? (Siegel 1989, 39)."

According to the story, Kaldi's curiosity got the better of him, and he decided to taste some of the red berries for himself. So it was that a simple goatherd discovered coffee and its invigorating and stimulating effects.

This popular tale, handed down in the guise of a legend, reflects a truth about the tendency of goats to deliberately nibble coffee berries for the stimulating effects they induce. These days such behavior is held strictly in check by farmers, who are extremely careful not to let domestic goats wreak havoc in their coffee plantations. And since both wild goats and wild coffee plants have all but disappeared, chances to observe the animals' "speedy" behavior have become increasingly rare.

In Ethiopia and Yemen, however, goats still go wild for khat (*Catha edulis*, from the family of Celastraceae), a plant with euphoric and stimulant properties chewed on a daily basis by millions of human inhabitants of those regions. The heavenly effects of this shrub, aptly called "flower of paradise," seem also to have been discovered by humans through herders' intimate connections with their flocks of goats. One Yemenite tale relates that the legendary goatherd Awzulkernayien noticed one of his animals wandering off from the herd one day and later running back to rejoin it with unprecedented swiftness. Awzulkernayien observed his doe goat's strange behavior for several days in a row until his curiosity was so piqued that he followed her. He discovered that she was wandering off from the others to nibble on the leaves and buds of a khat bush. Deciding to try them himself, he discovered their euphoric and rejuvenating effects and from that day forth never ceased to chew them.

Modern cultivators of khat are well aware that if a goat is given the chance to approach and browse on the flower of paradise, it will cease feeding on other plants altogether and will charge, butt, and kick anyone who tries to separate it from its "heaven."

The red bean or mescal bean—actually the seed of the leguminous evergreen shrub *Sophora secundiflora*—is a famous hallucinogen that has been used since antiquity by some tribes of Plains Indians in the course of their religious ceremonies. It is an extremely dangerous drug, however, containing cytisine and other alkaloids similar to nicotine; improper dosage can swiftly prove fatal. Perhaps for this reason, it was eventually supplanted in ceremonial use by the safer and more visionary peyote cactus. Archeological findings point to a continuity of use of *Sophora secundiflora* dating back at least 9000 years. Anthropologists suggest that Native Americans may have discovered its hallucinogenic effects by observing the bizarre behavior of animals who fed on it.

Siegel reports: "When I borrowed several goats from a nearby ranch and allowed them to graze near the red bean shrubs, I observed that a few goats were doing the same thing—trembling, falling, arising, and later browsing the plant again. They continued to fall and rise throughout the day, Mexican jumping beans in the hot Texas sun. Later I found that the hard-coated red beans that passed into their droppings were bruised sufficiently to allow for a partial release of the alkaloids. . . . It was getting dark and time for the animals to rest when I saw that the affected goats isolated themselves from the others. Meanwhile, my packhorses had already discovered the shrubs and were busily tearing into them. I rushed to pull them away. They reared and bucked with excitement. I managed to tie all but one of them to a safe tree. He ran to a nearby hill where he stayed all night, continually walking and tossing his head. At daybreak I awoke to find him back at the red bean shrub. . . . I was astonished by this persistence for intoxication (Siegel 1989, 55–56)."

6

BIRDS ON a BINGe

The most famous example of collective drunkenness in birds is that of American robins during their annual February migration to California, and in particular to the small town of Pleasant Hill. The amazing behavior of these birds on their arrival first made news in the 1930s.

Once they reach California, flocks of thousands of robins (the species *Turdus migratorius*) perch on small ornamental trees popularly known as California holly, though the Native Americans of the region call this scarlet fruit *toyon*. At this time of year the trees are laden with scarlet fruits called Christmas or holly berries. The robins, and other kinds of birds as well, gorge themselves on these fruits, bingeing until they are blatantly drunk. For about three weeks this region unintentionally hosts what can only be called a drunken orgy on the part of the birds, who become disoriented and confused, engaging in silly games with each other and fluttering wildly into cars and houses.

Ronald K. Siegel, who has studied this phenomenon with great attention, notes that although four or five holly berries would suffice to make a full meal, a single robin will gobble down as many as thirty at a time. Clearly the purpose of such gorging transcends simple nutrition; it would seem conclusive that the birds recognize and remember the fruit and seek out the intoxication induced by eating massive doses of it. In his book *Intoxication: Life in Pursuit of Artificial Paradise,* Siegel describes the behavior of a flock of about three thousand American robins after their arrival in Pleasant Hill. Excerpts from his observations follow.

"They quickly work their way to the outermost branches which begin to sag under their collective weight. As the branches wobble, so do the birds and they [the birds] start falling. Four birds are staggering on the ground, unable to fly. . . . [Now] there are eighteen birds on the ground. Several are still grasping berries in their beaks. A lone starling pilfers a berry right out of the locked beak of a robin. . . . A group of birds on the start of another feeding frenzy flies directly into my head and body. . . . I am driving in low gear to the edge of the field. There are thumps against the roof, then a robin smashes into the windshield. . . . Several birds are stunned momentarily when they fly into the windows and sides of houses. On the side of the road I find four more birds that have been killed in collisions with cars. . . . I performed autopsies on the dead birds. [They] revealed that the stomach, and sometimes the throat, of *every* bird was full of toyon berries, accounting for approximately 5 percent of their total body weight. Neither the stomach contents nor the berries themselves showed evidence of fermentation or alcohol. . . . Death was caused by a massive trauma inflicted by the collisions, secondary to an unknown intoxication (Siegel 1989, 58–59)."

Apparently, then, there have been no true cases of overdose in the robins and other birds who get high on the holly berries, and the only fatalities — very few, statistically speaking — are due to the presence of human beings: their cars, windows, and random acts of brutality. The local press, which almost every year dedicates a paragraph or two to the bizarre behavior of the migrating robins, frequently refers to the deaths of birds who have flown into cars or houses as "suicides," a misnomer and completely erroneous interpretation of the facts.

During the same time period and in the same region of California, birds become intoxicated on the fruits of yet another shrub, *Pyracantha,* a member of the rose family popularly known as firethorn. In this case, the birds act "like winged clowns: flying, falling, and hopping about in the most erratic, albeit entertaining, ways. Some were found fluttering in the dirt with wings awry, teasing backyard cats. Others teetered on window ledges and pecked at their reflections. Because firethorns were often planted near homes and roads, collisions with windows and cars were reported more frequently than with toyon (Siegel 1989, 60)."

The bark of the toyon tree was used by the native tribes of California for tanning and its fruits were roasted and eaten or brewed to make an intoxicating cider. However, it is not yet known precisely which substances in these sour, scarlet fruits are responsible for their inebriant effects on birds *or* humans, who have sometimes experienced delirium and visions after drinking toyon cider. Possibly they are due to the presence of psychoactive saponins, since another case of collective drunken bird binges relates to Tartarian honeysuckle, a source of similar saponins. Tartarian honeysuckle,

Lonicera tatarica, is a shrub native to Asia but widely cultivated along the eastern coast of the United States. In this case as well, robins are the birds most attracted by its intoxicating berries.

In 1926 J. Grinnell observed the behavior of these birds in his garden: "There were dozens of robins on the bushes and everywhere on the ground. They appeared tame and dazed. Some lay on the earth in the dirt with their wings awry. I regretted the fact that their condition rendered the birds unusually easy to catch by our cat, who seemed to know very well that he could catch one any time he felt like it." This avian disruption peaks in June when the plant's berries are ripest and most colorful.

W. H. Bergtold added in his own report of 1930: "The inebriation of these birds has been observed in all its stages, from mild instability to a level of uncoordination sufficient to cause them to fall to the ground. It seems that some birds become utterly fearless and perhaps even a little belligerent, since they show no fear of passersby and curious spectators." Bergtold found it curious that the birds had not learned to avoid these berries, thus demolishing the belief that no animal will feed on harmful substances.

Siegel had the chance to observe birds engaged in some fascinating, even romantic behavior as he was watching a pair of cedar waxwings drunk on firethorn berries: "Despite their reputation for sleek plumage, never seeming to have a feather out of place, the waxwings were left rumpled and tipsy by the intoxications. Yet they still had the ability to engage in a unique courtship display. The male fluffed his feathers and turned his head away from the female, who did the same. Then the male passed a firethorn berry as a 'present.' He offered it to his partner at the tip of the beak and she accepted it. The berry was passed back and forth several times and, eventually, it was eaten by one of the birds at the end of the display.

"A courtship present stirs the romantic imagination. After all, love and addiction are often viewed as two sides of the same coin, or, for birds, the same berry (Siegel 1989, 60)."

For three years the ornithologist David McKelvey studied the pink pigeon *(Columba meyeri)*, native to the Mauritian islands and in danger of extinction despite the fact that it has evolved in the absence of predators. McKelvey concluded that the pink pigeon lives in intimate relationship with three different psychoactive plants: a species of *Aphloeia* called fandamon by the natives; a species of *Styllingia* of the family of Euphorbiaceae, known as fangam; and a species of *Lantana*. The pigeons feed on the berries of these three plants and get drunk, in which condition they become totally incapable of doing anything but wander around on the ground in a daze. When the British introduced the mongoose to the Mauritian islands, the pigeons were decimated by this formidable carnivore, which was probably astonished to find such a quantity of feathered prey unable to fly out of harm's way. The results of McKelvey's studies indicate that these particular psychoactive berries are physiological necessities to the pink pigeons; for this reason the birds tend to die in captivity, especially if they are taken away from their natural drugs (Kennedy 1987, 256).

Certain other bird species feed avidly on the seeds of the opium poppy and are notorious scourges of the great opium plantations.

Sparrows have been observed entering storehouses to feed on hemp seeds, which seem to excite and stimulate them. In fact, many kinds of birds show this partiality for marijuana seeds, and it is related in many different regions of the world that eating them modifies their behavior — that, for example, they "sing" at greater length and with more ardor and are more inclined toward amorous displays. People who raise parrots add a certain percentage of hemp seeds to their animals' diets to make them more talkative. In Italy many canary owners do the same thing, to stimulate their birds to sweeter song.

7
OTHER "OUT THERE" ANIMALS

In the Rocky Mountains of Canada, wild bighorn sheep will dare the gravest dangers, teetering precariously on knife-edged outcrops and ledges and scrambling down deep ravines to reach a certain lichen and devour it greedily, although its nutritional value is negligible. This slow-growing lichen, colored in vivid yellow and green, is found on the surface of rocks and boulders.

Young ewes frequently wander away from the group to seek out the lichen and consume it in great quantities. This behavior becomes such a stubbornly ingrained habit that the ewes, in their frenzied scraping at the rocks, wear their nipping teeth down to such a degree that they often lose them entirely. Local Native Americans found the probable explanation for this weird phenomenon when they discovered that the lichen was a narcotic—for sheep, goats, *and* human beings.

Baboons search for and feed on the red fruit of a tree from the family of Cycadaceae, a behavior not evidenced during times of famine, demonstrating that the consumption of this fruit is not for the purpose of nourishment. After eating this fruit they appear drunk, swaying when they walk and seemingly incapable of moving swiftly—so that they fall easy prey to human hunters. Fatalities directly linked to ingestion of this fruit have never been observed among baboons, although it is mortally poisonous to humans. Instead, the fruit appears to produce a pleasant sensation of euphoria in the animals, who have probably developed a tolerance to its poisonous effects (Marais 1940).

Australian koalas feed exclusively on the fresh leaves of the eucalyptus plant, a phenomenon well known to native aboriginal peoples as well as zoo curators all over the world. Also known is that this sole food source exerts a narcotic and relaxing effect on koalas; aboriginals believe that the animals are severely addicted. We are presented, to be sure, with an extreme case of double dependency involving all the members of a particular species, in which the elements of nutrition and drug use coincide completely.

Adaptation and habituation to eucalyptus leaves seems not to be genetically imprinted in koalas but to take place during the first few months of life through nursing and maternal education. This would seem to be proved by the fact that young koalas *have* been raised successfully on a different diet: cow's milk, bread, and honey. But crucial to this is immediate separation from the mother after birth.

There are countless cases in which the psychoactive properties of certain plants have been discovered by human beings through observation of animal behavior. In the forests of Gabon and the Congo, natives relate that they long ago noticed wild boars digging up and eating the hallucinogenic roots of the iboga bush (*Tabernanthe iboga,* of the family of Apocynaceae). In consequence, the boars become frenzied, leaping in every direction, displaying inexplicable fear reactions and suffering hallucinations. Porcupines and gorillas also *intentionally* feed on iboga for its effects. It was by observing and imitating these animals that natives deduced, and then experienced, the visionary properties of the plant.

In the course of my own researches in Gabon, which

explored the use of iboga in the Buiti religious cult practiced by the Fang, Mitsogho, Apindji, and other Bantu tribes inhabiting the equatorial forest, I was informed by many different people that various animal species also eat iboga to drug themselves. A Mitsogho shaman, or *nganga,* told me of iboga use among male mandrills. Mandrills live in widespread communities and adhere to a rigid hierarchical structure. At the top of the ladder is the alpha male, to whom other powerful males submit; these, in turn, dominate yet weaker males.

When a male mandrill must engage in combat with another, either to establish his claim to a female or to climb a rung of the hierarchical ladder, he does not begin to fight without forethought. Instead, he first finds and digs up an iboga bush, eating its root; next, he waits for its effect to hit him full force (which can take from one to two hours); and only then does he approach and attack the other male he wants to engage in battle. The fact that the mandrill *waits* like this to feel the full effect of the drug before attacking demonstrates a high level of premeditation and awareness of what he is doing.

The kava bush (*Piper methysticum,* of the family of Piperaceae) is scattered widely throughout the islands of Melanesia and Polynesia. Natives have long brewed an intoxicating beverage from its roots, which is still consumed by a large part of the population. Various tales regarding the original discovery of the special properties of kava mythologize some observation of the bizarre relation rats (*Rattus exculans*, to be exact) have to the plant. For instance, in one origin tale from the New Hebrides, a man watches again and again as a rat gnaws on the root of the kava, dies, and later returns to life. Finally the man decides to test the effects of the root on himself and in so doing instigates the people's use of kava. In fact, not only rats but also swine raid kava plantations to dig up and gnaw at the roots and are afterward clearly intoxicated (Samorini 1995a, 102).

Marijuana *(Cannabis)* growers must also contend with animals greedy for their harvest. In the Hawaiian islands, cows and horses must be guarded against, as they are particularly partial to the flowers of the plant. After browsing on them, these animals walk with a rolling, swaying gait. It was also thought for a while by growers on Maui that mongooses were responsible for the destructive raids on fields and warehouses where freshly harvested marijuana was kept because the seeds of the plant were often found in their scat. Ronald K. Siegel, who was called in to investigate, found it to be a surprising premise, as mongooses are such fierce carnivores that under certain conditions they will even kill and eat each other. Hoping to find an explanation for the presence of seeds in their stomachs, he set up time-lapse cameras in fields where mongoose scat had been located.

"*Rattus rattus*, or rats!" concluded Siegel. "Under the cover of darkness, rats mischievously stripped the plants for the seeds. At sunrise, a few stragglers, still feeding or perhaps slowed by intoxication, were quickly dispatched by the stealthy mongooses on their morning patrols. With lightning speed the mongooses would seize the rat by the top of the head and audibly crush the cranium. The mongooses ignored the marijuana; the seeds in their scat came from the breakfast rats (Siegel 1989, 153–54)."

In eastern Europe, lambs break into hemp fields, browse on the plants, and become "merry and mad." In the 1950s a veterinarian in Greece reported on the progress of a lamb that got high repeatedly on cannabis and that nevertheless developed and fattened perfectly normally (Cardassis 1951, 973).

In North America deer infiltrate hidden growing sites to graze on marijuana; in South America monkeys do the same.

Several years ago in California white-tailed rabbits were observed invading specialized gardens where the psychoactive cactus *Astrophytum myriostigma* was being grown. The rabbits seemed distinctly drunk after nibbling on these cactus plants. Once they sobered up, they returned to browse on the cacti again, becoming newly intoxicated (*Entheogen Review* 1998, 73).

Rats will feed on the fruit and aerial parts of *Ipomoea*

violacea (of the family of Convolvulaceae), popularly known as morning glory, but generally avoid ingesting its seeds, which contain elevated concentrations of certain psychoactive alkaloids also found in ergot. These seeds have been sought after by humans since ancient times and are still prized for their hallucinogenic properties. Rats have been observed, on occasion, to swallow a seed — particularly during severe weather conditions — and to consequently experience a state of intoxication characterized by head twitching.

Siegel once observed a couple of Hawaiian mongooses ignore their usual diet of meat, eggs, and fruit to chew the seeds of some morning glories growing in their outdoor pen. The two animals twitched their heads and wandered in circles, then stayed still for several hours. In the following months, they ignored the seeds entirely. But when one of the mongooses died, its mate returned to the morning glories, chewed its seeds, and became intoxicated. Among the tribal peoples of Mexico, these seeds are often eaten for consolation in times of bereavement; perhaps the surviving mongoose was doing the same (Siegel 1989, 72).

8

INTOXICATED INSECTS

We indicated in preceding chapters that drugs are used by the lower orders of animals, such as insects and mollusks. This fact—that drug use is encountered in animals considered low on the evolutionary scale—is disconcerting to many ethologists and biologists, since the biological chasm between higher and lower orders has been generally considered enormous. This gap has been thought to include the structure and complexity of the nervous system.

Yet some species of moth with long, specialized proboscises are uniquely adapted to suck the nectar from the flowers of the datura, a plant of the Solanaceae family that is notoriously hallucinogenic for human beings. In Arizona the *Manduca quinquemaculata* moth lives on a diet of *Datura meteloides* nectar and in doing so contributes to the pollination of its flowers. Only after countless observations did researchers realize that these moths appeared to be drunk once they had sucked the nectar. Observation of their intoxicated behavior had slipped easily through the cracks—first because it occurs at night, when the datura opens the corollas of its blossoms, and second, because botanists and entomologists who take the trouble to spend their nights on the ground beside datura plants are primarily interested in identifying the pollinating insects and capturing them while they are still inside the flowers.

But some researchers reported that after the moths suck the nectar of several flowers, "They seem clumsy when they land on the flowers and often miss the target and fall onto the leaves or the soil. They right themselves slowly and awkwardly. When they take to flight again, their movements are erratic, as if they were confused. But the moths seem to like this effect and return to suck more nectar from those flowers (Grant and Grant 1983, 281)."

The nectar of this type of datura probably contains the same psychoactive alkaloids present in other parts of the plant, which is harvested by human beings for its hallucinogenic properties. The Grants hypothesize that this nectar, intoxicating as it is to the moths, may function as a kind of recompense offered by the plant to the insects that pollinate its flowers. Their resulting behavior, however, can prove extremely dangerous to the moths: to lie, even briefly, in a daze on the ground or to fly slowly and awkwardly is also to fall easy prey to avid predators—other nocturnal insects, reptiles, and amphibians—that have learned to wait under the datura plants for their complacent victims.

Similar behavior is evidenced by a certain kind of bee that visits the blossoms of the tropical American orchids *Catasetum, Cynoches, Stanhopea,* and *Gongora,* which instead of nourishment produce liquid perfume. *Eulaema, Euplusia,* and *Euglossa* bees carve scratches into the flowers of these orchids, through which the liquid perfume seeps out. The bees then absorb it through their hind feet. These insects return time and again to the scratches they have cut in the flowers and are consequently clumsy in their movements, which has been interpreted to be the result of a narcosis (Dodson 1962). Other kinds of bees become inebriated after drinking the nectar of certain specialized Umbelliferae flowers. This particular relationship between insects and flowers, in which the plants reward their pollinators with a drug, is probably much more widespread than has heretofore been thought.

The chemist Paul Lindner (1923), an expert on fermentations, reported that the larva of the carpenter moth *(Cossus cossus)*, stag beetles, and squirrels all greedily drink the fermenting sap of oak trees and get drunk on this sort of natural beer.

Lennig writes of this that "stag beetles first begin to rustle and click; then they sway and fall off the tree, trying awkwardly to stand back up, now on one leg, now on another—rolling over onto their backs every time—and finally they yield to their drunkenness and sleep it off (Reko 1996, 182)."

Another drunkard in the insect kingdom is an enormous and extraordinarily beautiful butterfly, the *Charaxes jasius* (popularly known as the jasio or arbutus nymph), which lives in Italy, among other places, in groves of strawberry trees. The jasio has "tailed" wings and a horizontally silver-striped body. It is attracted by anything that ferments and produces alcohol, especially rotting fruits that have fallen to earth. To better observe this gorgeous lepidopteran, entomologists place small glasses of beer or wine in its immediate neighborhood. Before long the butterfly, attracted by the odor of alcohol, makes an appearance and hurls itself on the liquid to plunge its proboscis (a kind of tubular tongue kept rolled in its mouth, which, when unfurled, acts as a straw) into it. Proof that the jasio gets drunk on the alcohol it sucks up is provided by its subsequent slow and staggering flight (Delfini 1998).

Some species of ants host a particular kind of beetle in their colonies, providing it with food and care. In exchange, their guests allow the ants to lick secretions produced in the beetles' abdomens and released through two furry tufts called trichomes. According to Siegel, "the ants may become so overwhelmed by the intoxicating nature of these secretions that they become temporarily disoriented and less sure of their footing." Myrmecologists — entomologists who specialize in the study of ants — have only recently become aware of this strange relationship because of the modern observational instruments now available to them. In the case of the yellow ant, *Lasius flavus*, and the *Lomechusa* beetle, worker ants appear to become completely uninterested in their domestic tasks, instead devoting themselves exclusively, and for long periods of time, to sucking secretions from the beetles' abdomens. The ants also raise the beetles' larvae, cradling them in the incubating chambers constructed for those of their own species. In times of danger, when they must hastily carry the larvae to a safer place, they rescue the beetle larvae before they tend to their own. It is not rare to find hundreds of *Lomechusa* beetles lodged in a single ant colony, an imbalance that leads swiftly to low productivity and a ruinous decline of the colony as a whole.

Siegel says: "Excessive intake of the intoxicant can cause such mania in the colony that female ant larvae become damaged in such a way that they develop into useless cripples rather than reproductive queens. Accordingly, '*Lomechusa*-mania,' a case of severe addiction, can contribute to the decline and fall of the ant society (Siegel 1989, 73)."

9
the Lazarus fly: a new hypothesis

The curious relationship of certain moths to the flowers of the datura plant led me to reevaluate the singular behavior of the common housefly *(Musca domestica)* when presented with fly agaric, or *Amanita muscaria* (Samorini 1999). So long has this relationship been remarked on, that the very name of the mushroom derives from the Latin word for fly, *musca*.

Another common name for the fungus is fly-killer, since the insects that are so enticed by its cap fall "stone dead" after tasting it. For centuries, in fact, people have scattered fly agaric caps on their windowsills as an insecticide. To enhance their effect, they were often crushed and mixed in with a little milk or sugar; this not only attracted a larger number of flies but induced them to consume a greater quantity of the intoxicating substance. It appears that many flies perished from a simple case of overdose.

In fact, the victims of fly agaric all *appear* to have died, lying perfectly stiff on their backs with their legs folded up in the air. In reality, however, they have not died at all; if you leave them alone, you can come back in an hour or a day to find, surprisingly, that they have flown away. Of course, usually the "dead" flies are swept up and thrown out — or those that have woken up and flown off are replaced by others, indistinguishable from the first, who have come along later, become intoxicated, and fallen into a swoon — so the fact that they rise from the dead and go about their business has escaped general notice. Thus, popular belief has it that fly agaric is a fatal poison to flies. Yet even in centuries past there were mycologists and entomologists who realized that flies that had tasted the mushroom were only in a state of lethargy and who counseled people who used it as an insecticide to gather up the stupefied insects and throw them into the fire (examples are the French mycologists J. J. Paulet, writing in 1793, and F. S. Cordier, writing in 1870).

An attentive observer can watch the whole process of "death" and "resurrection." First, the flies perch on the cuticle of the mushroom cap and lick its surface. After five to twenty minutes some of them begin to manifest the symptoms of intoxication: their flight becomes erratic and uncoordinated; they stop buzzing and flitting around, and their movements slow down; then their wings begin to quiver and their legs to shake; and finally, they roll over onto their backs or one side with their legs in the air, completely immobile. If touched lightly with a pencil, some may react by sluggishly moving their legs while others remain unperturbed in their position. With the help of a magnifying glass, it is possible to observe the peristaltic movement of their bodies, however—clear proof that they are not dead. After a period of time that may vary from thirty minutes to fifty hours, the flies wake up. Shortly afterward they begin to engage in their normal activities and fly off as if nothing had happened.

Not all flies that come into contact with *Amanita muscaria* are equally intoxicated. Inebriation may depend on the length of time a given insect is exposed to the surface of the mushroom and seems to comprise different levels of intensity and manifestation, from unusually frenetic flight to the most complete catalepsy.

During the last half of the 1960's some collaborators of

the great French mycologist Roger Heim—one of the founding fathers of modern ethnomycology and a pioneer in the study of hallucinogenic mushrooms—undertook some experimental research at the Museum of Natural History in Paris, where Heim was director, on the relationship between the common housefly and fly agaric (Bazanté 1965–66; Locquin-Linard 1965–67). The purpose of their study was to determine the mushroom's level of toxicity for the fly, which tells us little about the relationship of the two in a natural state. The experi- menters' conditions were contrived, as they forced a certain number of flies to live in the restricted quarters of a petri dish in direct and prolonged contact with the fly agaric or a liquid extract of it. As a result, they observed a high mortality rate in the intoxicated insects. This may have been due to the phenomenon of overdose induced by the conditions of the experiment, or even—as was suggested by the researchers themselves—to the production by the mushroom of carbon dioxide, which kills flies by asphyxiation.

In the course of the same studies it was determined that the active principles of the mushroom affect the nervous, rather than the muscular, system of the insects and that they become intoxicated not only by the spores of fly agaric but also by those of *Amanita pantherina,* a very similar mushroom characterized by the same active principles and hallucinogenic properties as *Amanita muscaria.*

Other researchers (Bowden, Drysdale, and Mogey 1965) have shown that the flies' resuscitation begins with a return of move- ment, first to the legs and then to the wings. They have also discovered that the most actively intoxicant part of the fly agaric mushroom is the yellowish flesh directly beneath the red cuticle of its cap where the isoxazolic alkaloids that have proven hallucinogenic to human beings are located. At one time it was thought that the intoxicating agent for both flies and humans was the muscarine in fly agaric, but when pure muscarine was fed to the insects, they had no reaction to it at all. Demonstrably, the same alkaloids provide the "high" for both species.

There must be a reason, not attributable to random chance, for the flies' strange behavior. It is hardly likely that they should always have been attracted to and intoxicated by fly agaric—generally without dying from it—by sheer accident. We should keep in mind the philosophical maxim that chance, or rather what we consider to be chance, is usually nothing but a measure of our ignorance; when we are unable to identify cause and effect in events we observe, we tend to justify them by turning to the concept of random occurrence.

I began, then, to formulate a new hypothesis regarding the relationship in nature between fly agaric and flies, especially in light of all the other information I had been gathering on animals, including insects, that drug themselves. It is not a case, I propose, of poisoning suffered by careless flies attracted to the mushroom—a fairly inexplicable sort of intoxication, at best, since it would have to be attributed to an evolutionary "oversight" on the part of these insects—but of an act of *intentionality*, in which they seek the experience of becoming inebriated by the fungus. Their behavior is similar to that of the *Manduca* moths' with the datura flowers: the flies are drugging themselves on fly agaric.

In nature (as opposed to a petri dish), where they can enjoy an unconstrained relationship with their drug, not all flies that perch on the mushroom and lick it fall "stone dead," that is, into a state of catalepsy. Human beings who smoke cannabis undergo its physical and psychic effects not instantly but gradually, and these range from conditions of mental and physical stimulation (the so-called high) to ecstatic and visionary states accompanied by a physical sedation that grows ever more profound until it reaches total immobility, which may last for several hours. This variability of affect depends not only on dosage but also on individual tolerance and reaction, as well as on differing levels of personal evolution in relationship to the drug.

To return to our flies, then, it seems possible that what we have so far observed of their intoxicated behavior is only its most profound and evident extreme—the only phase of it, in fact, that is evident to us at all. It is quite probable that the many flies who come into contact with the fly agaric mushroom without falling into a state of paralysis are nonetheless experiencing various stages of inebriation.

The scientist A. Morgan wrote, after observing a fruit fly *(Drosophila)* under the influence of a "lick" of fly agaric: "It tried to fly away and fell in spirals onto the table where the mushrooms were set out. It remained motionless for at least a minute, seemingly dead; then it collected itself and flew off (Morgan 1995, 102)." So probably not only the common housefly but an entire group of insects — particularly those whose habitat is the undergrowth — considers fly agaric to be its own, absolutely natural paradise.

But there is more to this story. Our new hypothesis might explain, in ecological terms, the universal and age-old symbolic relationship between fly agaric and toads.

In English and in various Eurasian languages the fly-agaric mushroom is commonly known as a toadstool. Most modern ethnomycologists have accepted the widespread interpretation that this is a simple semantic association due to the toxicity of both toads and fly agaric. J. Ramsbottom relates, in *Mushrooms and Toadstools*, the popular belief that these mushrooms "are made of poisonous substances in the soil and the poison of toads, and that they always grow in places where toads abound, giving shelter to these creatures (Ramsbottom 1953, 3)."

We know very little as yet about the intimate relationships between different species in their natural habitats. An example of our profound ignorance is scientists' recent and surprising discovery about the nature of moths' attraction to datura. In all my encounters with fly agaric in the Alpine woods, I have seen toads *(Bufo bufo)* in its vicinity only a couple of times. But I have to admit that I've never *looked* for them in those wide areas of underbrush scattered with "toadstools," nor have I lingered for long among these mushrooms, which can easily disseminate more than a hundred carpophores throughout the underbrush, covering the forest floor beneath dozens of trees.

Toads eat larvae and slow-moving insects. It is difficult for them to catch flies unless the flies are moving more slowly than usual for some reason—if they are wounded, for example, or if they are *drunk.*

Thus it is possible to formulate the following hypothesis: Given that flies are attracted by fly agaric and that when they are intoxicated by it their movements slow down to the point of paralysis, toads may have *learned* this and may, when they come across one of these mushrooms, sit under or nearby it and wait for easy prey, just as the predators of the moths wait for them to fall into their mouths beneath the datura blooms.

10
aNimaLs, HumaNs, aND DRuCs: tHe wHy of it aLL

In an essay written in 1890 and entitled "Why Do Men Stupefy Themselves?" the Russian author Leo Tolstoy described human drug use as a means of escaping from the self: "The cause of the worldwide consumption ption of hashish, opium, wine, and tobacco lies not in the taste, nor in any pleasure, recreation, or mirth they afford, but simply in man's need to hide from himself the demands of conscience (Tolstoy 1988)."

This kind of explanation has been the rallying cry of the most fundamentalist prohibitions. Although there are, without a doubt, those who drown their regrets in wine and numb themselves on the most disparate drugs to escape reality, today we know that the reasons behind the use of psychoactive substances are much more complex than this and that they are associated with the universal phenomenon of altered states of consciousness.

Drug use, like many other human behaviors, is dictated by the search for pleasure, which does not necessarily conceal within itself that need to hide from oneself attributed to it by Tolstoy; pleasure seeking is an instinctive behavior intrinsic to all humanity, and only its excesses acquire pathological characteristics. Moralistic ideologies tend to identify the search for pleasure with its pathological forms, just as they equate the phenomenon of drug use with the "drug problem." Human beings tend to try to modify their ordinary state of consciousness by the most disparate means to experience life in other altered mental states. This atavistic human behavior can be considered a behavioral constant. It is an impulse that manifests itself in human society without distinction of race or culture; it is completely cross-cultural (Samorini 1995a).

The alteration of states of consciousness, subject of a specific science (cf. Tart 1977), aside from occurring spontaneously, can be achieved by means of a wide spectrum of techniques, which people have gradually discovered and drawn upon in the course of human history. These range from sensory deprivation, bodily mortification, meditation, and asceticism to techniques that depend on dance or the sounds of particular musical instruments to trigger states of trance and possession, and include—last but certainly not least—methods based on the use of drugs extracted from plants with psychoactive properties.

This last is one of the most ancient of all techniques for the modification of consciousness. Archeological data confirm that it was already practiced in the Stone Age, a fact that might lead us to the conclusion that it originated in that archaic chapter of human history.

A more logical deduction, however, now that we have discovered its widespread existence in the animal kingdom, is that drug-induced alteration of consciousness *preceded* the origin of humans. Drugging oneself is a behavior that reaches across the entire process of animal evolution, from insects to mammals to women and men.

Today our knowledge is much greater than that avaliable to Tolstoy, at least regarding the history of drugs and the strict relationship that has always existed and continues to exist between their use and the intellectual, religious, and spiritual spheres of human activity.

The science of drugs came into being in the nineteenth century. One of its founding fathers, the Italian Paolo

Mantegazza (a contemporary of Tolstoy's but much more knowledgeable about the phenomenon than the Russian writer), intuited the universality and inevitability of this human behavior and the importance of studying it by taking a scientific approach. "All this, in a not-too-distant future, will be a great science," he wrote in one of his voluminous treatises on drugs, adding that "the aesthetics of the nourishments of the nervous system will continue to grow indefinitely and untiringly, until no one on our planet will be able to crush it underfoot (Mantegazza 1871, 2:680; cf. Samorini 1995b)."

In his search for the reasons that drive men to drug themselves, Tolstoy observed only that which is a *degeneration* of this human behavior, the fruit of modern society and its conflicts. Using drugs to escape reality and one's own conscience is not the rule but the exception, and its malignant growth is due to the widespread neurosis of modern society.

Historically speaking, the fundamental motive for using drugs springs from a desire to understand reality more fully, not to escape it. Many human cultures have placed some drug, held to be sacred, at the center of their religious paradigms, considering it the fulcrum of their systems of interpretation of various aspects of life and reality. Used under appropriate conditions—that is, in particular environmental and psychological settings—

drugs induce experiences accompanied by profound emotional and intuitive states that can be illuminating and revelatory. The elaboration and interpretation of these experiences contribute to the development of both individual and societal interpretations of reality.

The search for knowledge and the search for pleasure: these are the basic motivations behind the universal human use of drugs. Inappropriate approaches to and ignorance about drugs can lead to behaviors interpretable as the need to hide from oneself, as described by Tolstoy. Yet even in these cases, which we may define as pathological, we must exercise care in the expression of judgments with purely moralistic connotations. A new theory has recently found widespread acceptance among scholars and workers in the field of addiction: the theory of self-medication. According to this hypothesis, the heroin addict could well be a person in whom the production of endorphins—opiate substances produced naturally by the body—is lower than average. This individual may be finding a solution, more or less unconsciously, to his or her neurochemical imbalance by taking an exogenous opiate: heroin.

To follow a different line of thought, human drug use might have an adaptive function in relationship to surrounding reality. In fact, some modern sociologists and anthropologists have directly denominated drugs with the term *adaptogens*, that is, substances that facilitate adaptation to the surrounding environment, whether that be a village of huts immersed in the Amazonian rain forest or a frustrating and neurosis-ridden Western city.

Joseph M. Fericgla, who studied the use of the hallucinogenic beverage ayahuasca among the Shuar of Ecuador, wrote: "Ethnographic data oblige us to accept that one of the ends that explicitly induce human beings to consume *ayahuasca* (and by extension, hallucinogens in general) exists in relation with certain cognitive processes which allow for improvement in adaptive efficacy. In summary, we can state that *ayahuasca* is used traditionally to activate compensatory mechanisms of conduct, applied to self-analysis and the search for resolution to presenting conflicts, whether emotional in character or adaptive in general; it serves as an emotive accelerator with a cathartic resolution (Fericgla 1996, 5)."

In both hypotheses—self-medication, with its purely medical connotation, and adaptogenic function, with its psychological and sociological connotations—we are confronted with new interpretations of human drug use that, although not yet fully developed, are at least free of the stinging distortions of moralistic prejudice. They are *scientific* hypotheses.

Now, by turning our attention to the animals that drug themselves in nature, we can draw some further deductions. I will put forth, first of all, a suggestion and a further hypothesis: that natural drug-using behavior may be much more widespread in the animal world than that which we have so far discerned. In other words, it would seem that we are only at the beginning of this knowledge. And the phenomenon of animals that drug themselves becomes ever more important as it leads us to a fuller comprehension of the motivations that induce human beings to do the same.

It is difficult to reason in terms of animals' states of consciousness. Anthropocentric as we are, we are used to negating any form of consciousness at all in other species, especially in the lower orders of animals. Orthodox scientific thought is permeated by the philosophical dogma known as behaviorism, which excludes the possibility of thought of any kind in the animal kingdom.

When we speak of conscious thought, we generally divide it into two principal modes of consciousness: perceptive consciousness, which is essentially conscious perception and which may comprise memories or thoughts directed toward objects or events as well as immediate sensory information, and reflective consciousness, which implies a form of introspection—that is, thinking about one's own thoughts themselves.

Studies of animal behavior are providing ever more data in direct contradiction to behaviorism's rejection of animal mentality, and more and more scholars and researchers are distancing themselves from the behavioristic paradigm and beginning to admit the possibility of perceptive consciousness in animals. They are coming up with evidence that animals can, at the very least, process simple forms of thought (Griffin 1999). The phenomenon of animals that drug themselves provides confirmation for this hypothesis.

It is difficult to comprehend what animals *feel* when they drug themselves. In certain cases it would seem clear that they experience sensory hallucinations, but this is not enough in itself to understand their drugged condition in its complexity. The same holds true for human beings. The hallucinations a person is subject to under the influence of a hallucinogen are, by and large, only marginal products of the whole experience and are interpreted as such by the experimenters themselves. The contents and sense of a human psychedelic experience reach far beyond the visual and auditory hallucinations that accompany them. We must therefore take care not to judge the state of a drugged animal solely by its hallucinatory component.

The best we can do for the moment is to humbly acknowledge our ignorance and seek to be as open as possible and as free from the moral dogmas and presumptions that afflict our species as we can. The fact that a human behavior such as drug use, so insistently denigrated and prohibited because it is considered unnatural and therefore immoral, is also to be found in the rest of nature and practiced by many animals should teach us to be more cautious in our evaluations and convictions.

Ronald K. Siegel, the only scholar so far to have shown interest in this question, as well as having the courage to confront it head-on, concludes that the search for intoxication via drugs is a *primary motivational force* in the behavior of living beings. According to Siegel, data gathered up to this point demonstrate "that drug seeking and drug taking are biologically normal behaviors. . . . The ability of a drug to serve as a reward or reinforcer for behavior is not dependent on any abnormalities in the brain. Rather, those drugs that animals select to use are those capable of interacting with the normal brain mechanisms developed through evolution to mediate biologically essential behaviors directed toward food, water, and sex. In a sense, pursuit of intoxicating drugs is the rule rather than an aberration (Siegel 1989, 100)." Taking it even further, Siegel reaches the conclusion that intoxication, in animals as in human beings, has "adaptive evolutionary value (ibid., 211)."

I arrived long ago at the same conclusions, though my path wound through somewhat different conjectures than Siegel's. In one of my early works I underlined the import- ance of a certain biological concept: the "Provocative

Operation (PO) factor" or, "depatterning factor" as defined
and analyzed by the American doctor Edward De Bono
during the 1960s.

Referring specifically to the human mind and its
thought processes, De Bono defines the PO factor as that
fundamental function whose purpose is to act as a
"depatterning" tool to "throw consolidated models into
disorder." PO is an antiverbal concept: "The function of
language is to reinforce existing models; the function of
PO is to facilitate escape from these models (De Bono
1965, 208)." The depatterning factor shares strong
similarities with humor and intuition in the human mind.
Like both humor and intuition, "PO gives a person
permission to use ideas that are not coherent with
experience. With PO, rather than rejecting these ideas, a
person can use them as springboards toward other ideas.
PO therefore allows for the use of 'intermediate
impossibilities.' Since these 'impossible' ideas do not fit
established models, they render possible a certain distance
from existential experience. PO is a liberating device that
frees [the mind] of the rigidity of established ideas,
schemes, divisions, categories and classifications. PO is
an instrument for insight (De Bono 1969, 246–65)."

In my own considerations, I added that "PO heightens
the level of uncertainty and therefore the possibilities of
finding new mental pathways; it augments its own

entropy," and noted the strict similarities between De Bono's depatterning factor and the effects of LSD and hallucinogens in general (Samorini 1981).

The depatterning factor that De Bono discovered in the human mind could well be a function specific to all living beings. All living species are characterized by a few primary functions, such as nutrition and reproduction, which are indispensable to their preservation. But these alone are not enough; for the species to be able to preserve itself over time it must include the capacity to evolve, adapting and modifying itself in response to continual environmental changes. The principle of conservation (of that which has been acquired) tends to rigidly preserve established schemes and patterns, but modification (the search for new pathways) requires a depatterning instrument, or function, capable of opposing — at least at certain determined moments — the principle of conservation. It is my impression that drug-seeking and drug-taking behavior, on the part of both humans and animals, enjoys an intimate connection with the factor PO depatterning.

Since it is almost always only a certain percentage of members of any given species that engages in such behavior, this percentage may perform a depatterning function not only for itself but for the species as a whole.

Returning to the human arena, we must take into account the fact that all human behaviors, including the primary functions of nutrition and reproduction, are mediated by *culture*.

Having identified a *natural* component in the human impulse to take drugs—by observing the same impulse made manifest in the animal kingdom—the problems linked to human drug use must be found in the *cultural* component that mediates this behavior. In other words, the *drug phenomenon* is a natural phenomenon, while the *drug problem* is a cultural problem.

The development of new, amoral interpretations of the drug phenomenon is very recent; like all dawning ideas, they are still imperfect and imprecise. Yet given time and mental space, an open-minded approach, they will coalesce into a more complete formulation, which will bring us ever closer to a true theory of drugs, to a more mature paradigm than Leo Tolstoy's.

The drug problem in modern society is not so much due to the existence of drugs or the natural impulse to take them as to the deculturization of the human approach to them. To ensure that human drug use does not debase itself and become "bestial," it is important that it, like all other human behaviors, be mediated by appropriate cultural understanding and knowledge. Depriving the individual and his or her society of this knowledge—an understanding, above all, of *how* to use drugs and in which contexts their use is appropriate—paves the way for improper approach and use and, consequently, for the drug problem.

Tangible improvement of the drug problem can only come about by means of scientific study of the drug phenomenon and identification of the variables that regulate this phenomenon in the context of the intimate relationship between nature and human culture.

References

Abel, O. 1923. Amerikafahrt. Jena, Germany: G. Fischer.

Bazanté, G. 1965–66. Un problème à éclaircir: celui de la tue-mouche. L'Amanite tue-mouche, bien ou bien mal nommée? Revue de Mycologie 30:116–21; 31:261–68.

Bergtold, W. H. 1930. Intoxicated robins. *Auk* 47:571.

Bowden, K., A. C. Drysdale, and G. A. Mogey. 1965. Constituents of *Amanita muscaria*. *Nature* 206:1359–60.

Camporesi, P. 1980. *Il pane selvaggio*. Bologna: Il Mulino.

Cardassis, J. 1951. Intoxication des Équidés par Cannabis indica. Recueils de Médicine Vétérinaire 127:971–73.

Celli, G. 1999. *Vita segreta degli animali*. Casale Monferrato, Italy: Piemme.

Cordier, F. S. 1870. *Les champignons de France*. Paris: Rothschild.

De Bono, E. 1965. Il cervello e il pensiero. In *Il cervello: Organizazzione e funzioni*, AA.VV. Milan: Le Scienze, 203–208.

———. 1969. *The Mechanism of mind*. New York: Penguin

Delfini, M. 1998. *La vita segreta degli insetti geniali*. Padua: Muzzio.

Dodson, C. H. 1962. The importance of pollination in the evolution of the orchids of tropical America. *Bulletin of the American Orchids Society* 31:525–34, 641–49, 731–35.

Entheogen Review. 1998. 7(3): 73.

Fericgla, J. M. 1994. Alucinógenos o adaptógenos inespecíficos? In *Plantas, Chamanismo y Estados de Consciencia.* AA.VV. Barcellona: Los Libros de la Liebre de Marzo, 231–52.

————. 1996. Teoria e applicazioni dell'immaginazione generata dall'ayahuasca. *Eleusis* 5:3–18.).

Floru, L., J. Ishay, and S. Gitter. 1969. Influence of psychotropic substances on hornet behaviour in colonies of *Vespa orientalis* F. (Hymenoptera). *Psychopharmacology* 14:323–41.

Grant, V., and K. A. Grant. 1983. Behavior of hawkmoths on flowers of *Datura meteloides. Botanical Gazette* 144: 280–84.

Griffin, D. R. 1999. *Menti animali.* Turin, Italy: Boringhieri. Originally published in English as *Animal minds.* (Chicago: University of Chicago Press, 1992).

Grinnell, J. 1926. Doped robins. *Condor* 28:97.

Harney, J. W., J.D. Leary, and I.B. Barofsky. 1974. Behavioral activity of catnip and its constituents: nepetalic acid and nepetalactone. *Federal Proceedings* 33:481.

Kennedy, A. B. 1987. Ecce *Bufo*: il rospo in natura e nell'iconografia degli Olmec. *Quaderni di Semantica* 8: 229–63. Originally published in English as The toad in nature and in Olmec iconography. *Current Anthropology* 23 (1982): 273–90.

Lewin, L. 1981 [1924]. *Phantastika.* 3 vols. Milan: Savelli.

Lilly, J. C. 1981. *La comunicazione tra l'uomo e il delfino.* Rome: Cesco Ciapanna.

Lindner, P. 1923. *Entdeckte Verborgentieten.* Berlin.

Locquin-Linard, M. 1965–67. Ètude de l'action de l'*Amanita muscaria* sur le mouches. *Revue de Mycologie* 30: 122–23; 31:269–76; 32:428–37.

REFERENCES

Mantegazza, P. 1871. *Quadri della natura umana: Feste ed ebbrezze.* 2 vols. Milan: Brigola.

Marais, E. 1940. *My friends the baboons.* New York: McBride.

McGowan, C. 1999. *Predatori e prede.* Milan: Longanesi. Originally published in English as *The Raptor and the Lamb.* (Armonk, N.Y.: Bafor International, 1997).

Molyneux, R. J., and L. F. James. 1982. Loco intoxication: Indolizidine alkaloids of spotted locoweed *(Astragalus lentiginosus). Science* 216:190–91.

Morgan, A. 1995. *Toads and toadstools.* Berkeley, Calif.: Celestial Arts.

Newton, P. N., and T. Nishida. 1991. Possible buccal administration of herbal drugs by wild chimpanzees, *Pan troglodytes. Animal Behaviour* 39:798–801.

Ott, J. 1996. *Pharmacotheon.* Kennewick, Wash.: Natural Products.

Pagani, S. 1993. *Funghetti.* Turin, Italy: Nautilus.

Palen, G. F., and G. V. Goddard. 1966. Catnip and oestrous behaviour in the cat. *Animal Behaviour* 14: 372–77.

Paulet, J. J. 1793. *Traité des champignons.* 2 vols. Paris.

Ramsbottom, J. 1953. *Mushrooms and toadstools.* London: Collins.

Reko, V. A. 1996 [1938]. *Magische Gifte.* Berlin: VWB.

Rodriguez, E., et al. 1985. Thiarubrine A, a bioactive constituent of *Aspilia* (Asteraceae) consumed by wild chimpanzees. *Experientia* 41:419–20.

Samorini, G. 1981. *Riflessioni Lisergiche.* Bologna: Flash

——— . 1993. Funghi allucinogeni italiani. *Annali del Museo Civico di Rovereto,* suppl. vol. 8:125–49.

——— . 1995a, *Gli allucinogeni nel mito: Racconti sulle origini delle piante psicoattive.* Turin, Italy: Nautilus

————. 1995b. Paolo Mantegazza (1831–1910): Italian pioneer in the studies on drugs. *Eleusis* 2:14–20.

————. 1999. Fly agaric, flies and toads: a new hypothesis. *The Entheogen Review* 8 (3): 85–89.

————. 2000. *Funghi allucinogeni: Studi etnomicologici.* Vicenza, Italy: Telesterion.

Siegel, R. 1989. *Intoxication: Life in Pursuit of Artificial Paradise.* New York: Dutton.

Stafford, P. 1979. *Enciclopedia psichedelica.* Rome: Cesco Ciapanna. Originally published in English as *Psychedelics Encyclopedia.* (Berkely, Calif.: Ronin, 1978)

Takemoto, T., and T. Nakajima. 1964. Isolation of the insecticidal constituent from *Tricholoma muscarium. Yakugaku Zasshi* 84:1183–85.

Tart, C. 1977. *Stati di coscienza.* Rome: Ubaldini.

Thorn, R. G., and G. L. Barron. 1984. Carnivorous mushrooms. *Science* 224:76–78.

Todd, N. B. 1962. Inheritance of the catnip response in domestic cats. *Journal of Heredity* 53:54–56.

Tolstoy, L. 1988. *Perch la gente si droga? e altri saggi su società, politica, religione.* Milan: Mondadori.

Valieri, R. 1887. *Sulla canapa nostrana e suoi preparati in sostituzione della* Cannabis indica. Naples: Tipografia dell'Unione.

INDEX

Adaptogens, 80
Alán, xii
Alchornea cordifolia, xii
Alchornea floribunda, xii
Alcohol, 5. *See also* Durian
  butterflies and, 65–66
  hedgehogs and, 31
  pachyderms and, 27
  slugs and, 31
  snails and, 31.
Amanita muscaria. See Fly agaric
Animal behavior. *See* Ethology
Animal awareness
  human awareness distinguished
    from, ix
Antiparasitics, xii
Ants, beetles and, 66–67
Aphrodisiac, xii
  beetles as, x
Asceticism, 78
Aspilia, leaves of, 15
Astragalus lambertii. See Locoweed
Astragalus mallissimus. See Locoweed
Astrophytum myriostigma. See Cactus
Ayahuasca, 7, 81

Baboons, 56
Balanites aegyptica, 16
Bees, orchids and, 64–65
Beetles

ants and, 66–67
as aphrodisiac, x
  Lomechusa, 66–67
  stag, 65
Berries, 11
  Birds. *See also* Canaries;
    Pigeons, pink; Robins;
    Sparrows
  firethorn and, 51–53
  Tartarian honeysuckle and,
    51–52
Boars, iboga bush, 57
Bodily mortification, 78
Borassus (palm trees)
  pachyderms and, 27
Bufo bufo, 75. *See also* Toads
Butterflies, alcohol and, 65–66

Cactus, rabbits and, 60
Caffeine, spider webs and, 13
Canaries, hemp seeds and, 54
Canines, psilocybin mushrooms
  and, 41
Cannabis. See Marijuana
Caribou, fly agaric and, 40
Carpenter moth, 65
Cat civet, x
Catalepsy, 73
Catasetum orchid, 64
Catha edulis (khat), 45

93

Catnip, 4, 32–36, viii
Cats. *See* Felines
Chachaquilia. See Locoweed
Charaxes jasius. See Butterflies
Chipmunks, fly agaric and, 40
Cigarettes, smoking tobacco, viii, 9
   addiction to, 6
Cocaine, forced administration
   of, 10
Cod liver oil, x
Coffee berries, goats and, 43–47
Columba meyeri. See Pink pigeon
Consciousness, 82
   alteration of, 76–78
Cossus cossus. See Carpenter moth
Cows
   locoweed and, 19
   marijuana and, 59–60
Cultural environment, effects of
   drugs on, 7, 87–88
Cycadaceae, 56
Cynoches orchid, 64
Cystium diphysum. See Locoweed

Datura flower, nectar of, 11
   moths and, 63–64, 73
Datura meteloides. See Datura flower,
   nectar of
Deconditioning, ix
Deer
   marijuana and, 60
   musk, x
"Dewatering factor," 85–86
Deschematizzazione, ix
Dogs. *See* Canines
Dolphins, LSD and, 14
Donkeys, addiction to locoweed, 19
Dream fish, x
Drosophilia. See Fruit flies
Drug(s), animals and, 1–17
   accidental ingestion of, 10–12
   addiction to, 2
   of animal origin, x

cultures and, 79–80
   definition of, 4–6
   effects of, 7
   feelings of, 83
   forced administration of, 9–10
   intentional ingestion of, 10–12
   intentions of animals and, 8
   medicine and, x
   laboratory, 9–10
   phenomenon, 87
   psychoactive substances used
     by, x
   state of consciousness and, 82
Drug(s), humans and, 76–88,
   76–88. *See also* Plants, drug
   cannabis, 73
   fundamental motive of, 79–80
   plants' use by, ix
   pleasure and, 77, 80
   problem, 87–88
   self-medication and, 81
   sources of, viii
   state of consciousness and,
     76–78
   types of, 12–13
   urge to take, 79
Drugged, 7–8
Durian, 29
   elephants and, 29
   flying foxes and, 29
   monkeys and, 29–30
Durio zibethinus. See Durian

Elephants, 27–30
   calves of, 28–29
   durian *(Durio zibethinus)*
     and, 29
   fermented fruits and, 27–30
Ethnobotany, ix, x
Ethnopharmacognosy, ix
Ethnozöopharmacognosy, x
Ethology, viii, ix
Eucalyptus, koalas and, 56–57

Euglossa bee. *See* Bee
Eulaema bee. *See* Bee
Euplusia bee. *See* Bee
Ewes, lichen and, 56

Felines, 32–37
  catnip and, 32–36
  Japanese cats, matatabi and, 37
  purgative grasses and, x, 15
  valerian and, 36–37
Fermented fruits, elephants and,
  27–30
Firethorn, 51–53
Fly agaric mushrooms, 11. *See also*
  Housefly, fly agaric and
  caribou and, 40
  chipmunk and, 40
  found in urine, 39–40
  housefly and, 68–75
  reindeer and, 38–40
  squirrel and, 40
  toadstools and, 74–75
Flying foxes
  durian *(Durio zibethinus)*
    and, 29
Fruit flies, 74

Garbancillo. See Locoweed
Goats
  coffee berries and, 43–47
  lichen and, 56
  psilocybin mushrooms and,
    41, 42
Gongora orchid, 64
Gorillas, iboga bush and, 57
Grass, crazy. *See* Locoweed
Grasses, purgative, x, 15

Hallucinogenic drugs
  lysergic acid diethylamide
    (LSD), 6, 13–14, 86
  mushrooms, 38–39, 40–42
  psilocybin mushrooms, 40

sophora secundiflora and,
  45–46
Hashish, spider webs and, 13
Hedgehogs, alcohol and, 31
Heim, Roger, 71
Hemp seeds. *See also* Marijuana
  canaries and, 54
  lambs and, 60
  parrots and, 54
  sparrows and, 54
Hens, addiction to locoweed, 19
Herbs. *See* Felines
Heroin, forced administration
  of, 10
Holly berries, robins and, 49–50
Honey, toxic, x
Honeysuckle, Tartarian, 51–52
Hormones, x
Hornets, LSD and, 13–14
Horses
  addiction to locoweed, 19
  marijuana and, 59–60
Housefly, fly agaric and, 68–75
  catalepsy in, 73
  effect on nervous system, 71
  effects of, 69–70
  as insecticide, 69
  resuscitation in, 72
  toads and, 74–75
Huffman, Michael, xii
Human awareness
  animal awareness distinguished
    from, ix
Humans. *See* Drug(s), humans and

Iboga bush
  boars and, 57
  gorillas and, 57
  porcupines and, 57
Immunostimulating ants, x
Inebriation, deliberate seeking
  of, ix
Insects, 62–68

Intoxication, accidental, viii
Ipomoea violacea. See Morning
   glory

Japanese cats
   matatabi and, 37

Kava bush, 58–59
Khat (Catha edulis), 45
Koalas, eucalyptus and, 56–57

Lambs, hemp fields and, 60
Libidostimulant plant drugs, xii
Lichen, sheep and, 55–56
Lindner, Paul, 65
Locoweed, 18–26
   addiction to, 19
   antelopes and, 19
   death and, 23–24
   mules and, 19
   pigs and, 19
   rabbits and, 19
   sheep and, 19
Lomechusa beetle, 66–67
Lonicera tatarica, See Tartarian
   honeysuckle
LSD. See Lysergic acid
   diethylamide (LSD)
Lysergic acid diethylamide
   (LSD), 6, 86
   dolphins and, 14
   hornets and, 13–14
   spider webs and, 13

Mandrill, 58
Manduca quinquemaculata. See
   Moths
Mantegazzam, Paolo, 3
Mapacho, 7
Marijuana. See also Hemp seeds
   cows and, 59–60
   deer and, 60
   horses and, 59–60

monkeys and, 60
rats and, 59–60
Meditation, 78
Mescal plant, inebriant beans
   from, 11, 45
Miserotoxin, 25
Mongooses, morning glory and,
   61
Monkeys
   durian (Durio zibethinus) and,
   29–30
   marijuana and, 60
Morning glory
   mongooses and, 61
   rats and, 60–61
Moths
   carpenter, 65
   datura nectar and, 63–64, 73
Musca domestica. See Housefly
Muscular system
   fly agaric and, 71
Mushrooms, psilocybin, 40. See
   also Fly agaric
   canines and, 41
   goats and, 41–42

Nepeta cataria. See Catnip
Nepetalic acid, 35–36
Nervous system, drugs and, 5
   fly agaric and, 71
Nicotine, forced administration
   of, 10

Oak trees, fermenting sap of, 65
Opium poppy, 8–9, 54
Orchids, bees and, 64–65

Pachyderms, alcohol and, 27
Palm trees (Borassus),
   pachyderms and, 27
Pan troglodytes, 15
Panaeolus. See Mushrooms
Papio, 16

Parrots, hemp seeds and, 54
Pigeons, pink, 53–54
Piper methysticum. See Kava bush
Plants, drug
  human use of, ix
  libidostimulant, xii
  prosexual, xii
Porcupines, iboga bush and, 57
Prosexual plant drugs, xii
Provocative Operation (PO)
  factor, 85–86
Psilocybe semilanceata.
  See Mushrooms
Psychoactive substances, x
Psychoactive toad venom, x
Pyracantha. See Firethorn

Rabbits
  cactus and, 60
Rats *(rattus exculans)*
  kava bush and, 59
  marijuana and, 59–60
  morning glory and, 60–61
Red bean, 45
Reindeer, fly agaric and, 38–40
Robins, 48–51
  holly berries and, 49–50
  toyon and, 49

Samorini, Giorgio, ix, x
Seeds, crazy. *See* Locoweed
Self-medication, 80–81
Senses, enhanced, xi
Sensory deprivation, 78
Serum vaccines, x
Sheep
  lichen and, 55–56

Slugs, alcohol and, 31
Snails, alcohol and, 31
Sophora secundiflora, 45–46
Spanish fly, x
Sparrows, hemp seeds and, 54
Spider webs, LSD and, 13
Squirrels
  fly agaric and, 40
  sap of oak trees and, 65
Stag beetles, 65
Stanhopea orchid, 64
Stone Age, 78

Tabernanthe iboga, xii
Tabernanthe iboga. See Iboga bush
Tartarian honeysuckle, 51–52
Thiarubrine-A, 15
Tigers. *See* Felines
Toads, 74–75
Toadstool, fly agaric and, 74–75
Tobacco cigarettes, smoking, viii, 9
  addiction to, 6
Toyon, 49
Turdus migratorius. See Robins

Umbelliferae flower, 64
Urine, fly agaric found in, 39–40

Valerian, 36–37
Valieri, Raffaele, 36

Wasson, R. Gordon, ix

Zilla x notata, 13

BOOKS OF RELATED INTEREST

PLANTS OF THE GODS
Their Sacred, Healing, and Hallucinogenic Powers
by Richard Evans Schultes, Albert Hofmann, and Christian Rätsch

DMT: THE SPIRIT MOLECULE
A Doctor's Revolutionary Research into the Biology of
Near-Death and Mystical Experiences
by Rick Strassman, M.D.

ECSTASY: THE COMPLETE GUIDE
A Comprehensive Look at the Risks and Benefits of MDMA
Edited by Julie Holland, M.D.

MARIJUANA MEDICINE
A World Tour of the Healing and Visionary Powers
of Cannabis
by Christian Rätsch

A BRIEF HISTORY OF DRUGS
From the Stone Age to the Stoned Age
by Antonio Escohotado

ECSTATIC BODY POSTURES
An Alternate Reality Workbook
by Belinda Gore

ANIMAL VOICES
Telepathic Communication in the Web of Life
by Dawn Baumann Brunke

DOLPHINS AND THEIR POWER TO HEAL
by Amanda Cochrane and Karena Callen

Inner Traditions • Bear & Company
P.O. Box 388
Rochester, VT 05767
1-800-246-8648
www.InnerTraditions.com

Or contact your local bookseller